Amazing DIY Breathing Device

Breathing Retraining Manual

Artour Rakhimov

Dr. Artour Rakhimov

*"All chronic pain, suffering and diseases
are caused from a lack of oxygen at the cell level."*

**Arthur C. Guyton, The Textbook of Medical Physiology*, Fifth
Edition.**
* World's most widely used medical textbook of any kind
* World's best-selling physiology book

Disclaimer

Dr. Artour Rakhimov

TABLE OF CONTENTS

Introduction

Hundreds of medical studies have proved that when we breathe more than the medical norm (hyperventilate), we get less oxygen into our body cells. At the same time, virtually all chronic diseases are based on cellular hypoxia. All available research has also shown that sick people (heart disease, cancer, asthma, bronchitis, COPD, diabetes, and many other chronic conditions) breathe about 2-3 times more than the medical norm. Hence, the solution is to learn how to breathe less.

Dr. Konstantin Buteyko developed a method (the Buteyko breathing method) to normalize one's breathing pattern so that the person learns how to breathe less. As a result of breathing retraining, they experience relief from their symptoms and require less and less medication. Normalization of breathing, as Dr. Buteyko and about 200 his medical colleagues from the former USSR found, means normal body oxygenation and clinical remission of many chronic diseases.

I have been teaching the Buteyko method to hundreds of students, mostly in small groups, during the last 7 years. When Buteyko students improve their body oxygenation or CP (control pause), their health is indeed improved. Over 20 second CP means no symptoms and no medication for hypertension, asthma, bronchitis, and many other conditions. However, the main disadvantage of the Buteyko method is that very few people (less than 1% of the sick people) are able to learn the Buteyko breathing exercises from a book or manual.

Dr. Buteyko discovered this fact himself already in the 1960s and that is why he started to teach practitioners by choosing and training sick doctors.

This disadvantage (necessity of the practitioner or teacher) can be solved using a simple DIY breathing device. How? It is much easier to practice breathing exercises correctly using this DIY breathing device. Although, there are still restrictions, limits, and temporary contraindications, sick people can get a chance to have a better life, and this without learning it from a breathing teacher.

In 2009-2010, apart from teaching the Buteyko breathing exercises (reduced breathing) to groups, I also made numerous breathing devices for my students and explained to them how to use these devices. Weeks later I asked these students about their experiences and the efficiency of the DIY devices. The following facts were discovered:

1) My students were able increase their body oxygenation by as much as 5-15 seconds during one breathing session of about 15 minutes.

2) They got greater CP increases in comparison to Buteyko breathing exercises of the same duration.

3) They reported that it was much easier to practice with the device and they achieved more benefits from using the DIY breathing device.

4) However, when these students got up to 30-40 second CP, they usually preferred the reduced breathing exercises developed by Dr. K. Buteyko, since the Buteyko exercises do not require any device and can be practiced anywhere and/or at any time of the day, while being involved in other activities.

I still continue to teach both, the Buteyko breathing exercises and the use of the DIY breathing device, since each approach has its advantages. They greatly complement each other. Although I ask my students to practice both types of exercises during the course, I leave it up to my students to decide which exercises they want to practice after the course, this based on their own intuition, sensations, and recorded experience (their daily logs).

On average, for the initial stages of breathing retraining, the DIY breathing device is about 40-60% more efficient, in terms of CP (oxygenation) growth, than the typical session of Buteyko reduced breathing of the same duration. In addition, since it is easy to learn and practice, I have decided to share this idea with you.

Who can use this manual?

Normal breathing is a fundamental property of the healthy organism. Hence, breathing normalization is the natural way to deal with human body pathologies. While people with cardiovascular, lung, and some other problems require a different approach (see the next sections), this manual can and should be successfully used by people who suffer from any of these symptoms, disorders, and conditions and their combinations:

Bones, Joints & Muscles Conditions (arthritis; back & neck pain; Carpal tunnel syndrome; chronic fatigue syndrome & fibromyalgia; elbow pain (bursitis); knee pain; muscular dystrophies; osteoarthritis; osteochondrosis; osteoporosis; polyarthritis; rheumatoid arthritis / joint conditions; radiculitis (nerve root syndrome); scoliosis).

Brain & Nervous System (ADD/ADHD; addictions; alcoholism; Alzheimer's disease; anxiety; bipolar disorder; carpal tunnel syndrome; depression; dizziness; eating disorders; encephalitis; epilepsy; obsessive- compulsive disorder; meningitis (viral and bacterial); motor neurone disease, Parkinson's disease; phobias; post traumatic stress disorder (PTSD); schizophrenia; senile dementia, social anxiety disorder; vertigo) **Cancer** (stages 1 and 2; as an additional therapy for a standard complex treatment)

Eye disorders (cataracts; far-sightedness; glaucoma; macular degeneration)

Gastrointestinal problems (acute and chronic pancreatitis; cholecystitis; Crohn's disease; chronic gastritis; constipation; duodenal ulcer; gallstone disease; gastric ulcers; heartburn / GERD; hemochromatosis; IBS; IBD; liver cirrhosis; peptic ulcer; spastic colitis; weight loss)

Hormonal disorders (adrenal insufficiency; diabetes mellitus type 1; gestational diabetes; hyperthyroidism; hypothyroidism; prediabetes; reactive hyperglycemia and hypoglycemia; obesity)

Immune conditions (allergic conjunctivitis; allergies; dermatitis; hay fever; lupus; multiple chemical sensitivities)

Other conditions (anemia; cystic fibrosis; hemorrhoids; Raynaud's disease; thrombophlebitis; varicose veins)

Radiation disease

Sleep-related problems (bruxism, insomnia; restless leg syndrome; sleep apnoea; snoring)

Skin disorders (Acne; diathesis; eczema; psoriasis)

Upper respiratory disorders (sinusitis; rhinitis; adenoiditis; polyps; tonsillitis; laryngitis; pharyngitis; tracheitis and other related disorders

Urinary and kidney problems (pyelonephritis, glomerulonephritis, kidney stones; nephritis, nocturia; urinary incontinence; urinary tract infections)

Viral and bacterial conditions (AIDS (acquired immune deficiency syndrome); bird flu (Avian influenza); cellulitis (bacterial infection); cold; hepatitis A; hepatitis B; hepatitis C; influenza, Lyme disease; rubella (German measles); shingles; West Nile virus).

Women's conditions (cervical erosion; endometriosis; fibroids; fibromyomes; fibrotic mastopathy; irregularities of the menstrual cycle; menopause; sterility; toxicosis of pregnancy; yeast infections)

Note that it is impossible to provide a sensible classification of modern health problems ("diseases of civilization") due to overlaps and possible complex clinical pictures. The explanation for this is that modern medicine does not know the cause of these health problems. This manual suggests that all these conditions have one common cause. Hence, they are not separate disorders, but symptoms of one large disease, which we are going to investigate and address.

Who has special restrictions, limits, and temporary contraindications

Breathing retraining and breathing exercises produce a mild stress for the human body so that it can adapt to new conditions and function better in future. Such adaptive effects take place during, for example, physical exercise. It would be silly for an unfit person to try to run a marathon without rigorous preparation.

If the demands due to the exercises are too high, there is no adaptive response, and, as a result, the exercises can even produce a negative effect. Hence, breathing exercises should also be adjusted to the current adaptive abilities of the human organism. For example, people with existing cardiovascular and/or lung problems require certain modifications (individual tailoring) to their breathing retraining.

For example, a more gentle approach in relation to hypoxic and hypercapnic demands of breathing exercises (quick changes in air composition) is necessary for many patients with:
- **Heart disease** (aortic aneurysms; angina pectoris; arrhythmia; atherosclerosis (plaque buildup); cardiomyopathy; ciliary arhythmia (cardiac fibrillation); chest pain (angina pectoris); high cholesterol; chronic ischemia; congenital heart disease; congestive heart failure; coronary artery disease; endocarditis; extrasystole; heart murmurs; hypertension; hypertrophic cardiomyopathy; tachnycardia; pericarditis; postmyocardial infarction; stroke)
- **Migraine headaches and panic attacks**

Those people, who have existing problems with their lungs should avoid too fast and too large stretching (expansion or dilation) and shrinking (constriction) of their lungs. Hence, their inhalations and exhalations should be limited (not maximum) in their amplitude and

velocity. This relates to people with:
- **Respiratory disorders involving the lungs** (asthma, bronchitis, COPD, emphysema, cystic fibrosis, pneumonia, tuberculosis; pulmonary edema; etc.)

Other specific situations include:
- **Presence of transplanted organs**
- **Pregnancy**
- **Brain traumas**
- **Acute bleeding injuries**
- **Blood clots**
- **Acute stages (exacerbations) of life-threatening conditions (infarct, stroke, cardiac ischemia, etc.)**
- **Insulin-dependent diabetes (type 2 diabetes)**
- **Loss of CO2 sensitivity.**

If you suffer from any of these conditions, you should follow special suggestions (see below) due to restrictions, limits, and temporary contraindications.

Warning. *It is your responsibility, in cases of doubts to consult your family physician or GP about breathing retraining and use of this breathing device and manual for your specific health problems. And certainly consult your health care provider about any medication.*

1. What is wrong with the breathing of the sick?

1.1 Heart disease

Let us start with heart disease. Here are the results of 8 published independent medical studies about breathing rates (minute ventilation) in 8 groups of patients with heart disease. (The graphs are from the website.)

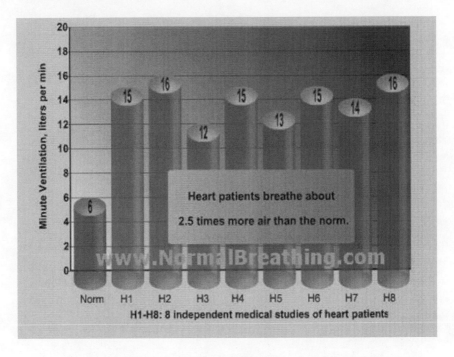

Table. Breathing rates in patients with heart disease.

*One row corresponds to one medical study/publication

Minute ventilation rates in heart patients			
Condition	Minute ventilation	Number of patients	References
Normal breathing	6 L/min	-	Medical textbooks
Healthy Subjects	6-7 L/min	>400	Results of 14 studies
Heart disease	15 (±4) L/min	22	Dimopoulou et al, 2001
Heart disease	16 (±2) L/min	11	Johnson et al, 2000
Heart disease	12 (±3) L/min	132	Fanfulla et al, 1998
Heart disease	15 (±4) L/min	55	Clark et al, 1997
Heart disease	13 (±4) L/min	15	Banning et al, 1995
Heart disease	15 (±4) L/min	88	Clark et al, 1995
Heart disease	14 (±2) L/min	30	Buller et al, 1990
Heart disease	16 (±6) L/min	20	Elborn et al, 1990

We can see that heart patients breathe too much. What is wrong with this?

If heart patients breathe more air than the medical norm, it is logical that their heart muscle gets less blood and oxygen supply (see explanation in the next section). Should these heart patients slow their breathing back to the norm, heart perfusion and oxygenation, state of blood vessels, and many other key parameters would again become normal. This would result in the disappearance of the symptoms of heart disease and no more need for medication.

References (in the same order)

Dimopoulou I, Tsintzas OK, Alivizatos PA, Tzelepis GE, Pattern of breathing during progressive exercise in chronic heart failure, Int J Cardiol. 2001 Dec; 81(2-3): p. 117-121.

Johnson BD, Beck KC, Olson LJ, O'Malley KA, Allison TG, Squires RW, Gau GT, Ventilatory constraints during exercise in patients with chronic heart failure, Chest 2000 Feb; 117(2): p. 321-332.

Fanfulla F, Mortara , Maestri R, Pinna GD, Bruschi C, Cobelli F, Rampulla C, The development of hyperventilation in patients with chronic heart failure and Cheyne-Stokes respiration, Chest 1998; 114; p. 1083-1090.

Clark AL, Volterrani M, Swan JW, Coats AJS, The increased ventilatory response to exercise in chronic heart failure: relation to pulmonary pathology, Heart 1997; 77: p.138-146.

Banning AP, Lewis NP, Northridge DB, Elbom JS, Henderson AH, Perfusion/ventilation mismatch during exercise in chronic heart failure: an investigation of circulatory determinants, Br Heart J 1995; 74: p.27-33.

Clark AL, Chua TP, Coats AJ, Anatomical dead space, ventilatory pattern, and exercise capacity in chronic heart failure, Br Heart J 1995 Oct; 74(4): p. 377-380.

Buller NP, Poole-Wilson PA, Mechanism of the increased ventilatory response to exercise in patients with chronic heart failure, Heart 1990; 63; p.281-283.

Elborn JS, Riley M, Stanford CF, Nicholls DP, The effects of flosequinan on submaximal exercise in patients with chronic cardiac failure, Br J Clin Pharmacol. 1990 May; 29(5): p.519-524.

1.2 Asthma

Let us look at MV (minute ventilation) in patients with asthma at rest. Here again, the breathing rates relate to the state of patients when they do not have any acute episodes or symptoms of their disease, since during exacerbations, chronically sick people breathe even more.

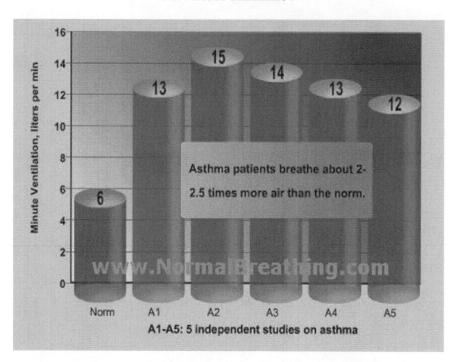

*One row corresponds to one medical study/publication

Minute ventilation rates in asthmatics			
Condition	Minute ventilation	Number of people	References
Normal breathing	6 L/min	-	Medical textbooks
Healthy Subjects	6-7 L/min	>400	Results of 14 studies
Asthma	13 (±2) L/min	16	Chalupa et al, 2004
Asthma	15 L/min	8	Johnson et al, 1995
Asthma	14 (±6) L/min	39	Bowler et al, 1998
Asthma	13 (±4) L/min	17	Kassabian et al, 1982
Asthma	12 L/min	101	McFadden & Lyons, 1968

References (in the same order)

Chalupa DC, Morrow PE, Oberdörster G, Utell MJ, Frampton MW, Ultrafine particle deposition in subjects with asthma, Environmental Health Perspectives 2004 Jun; 112(8): p.879-882.

Johnson BD, Scanlon PD, Beck KC, Regulation of ventilatory capacity during exercise in asthmatics, J Appl Physiol. 1995 Sep; 79(3): 892-901.

Bowler SD, Green A, Mitchell CA, Buteyko breathing techniques in asthma: a blinded randomised controlled trial, Med J of Australia 1998; 169: 575-578.

Kassabian J, Miller KD, Lavietes MH, Respiratory center output and ventilatory timing in patients with acute airway (asthma) and alveolar (pneumonia) disease, Chest 1982 May; 81(5): p.536-543.

McFadden ER & Lyons HA, Arterial-blood gases in asthma, The New Engl J of Med 1968 May 9, 278 (19): 1027-1032.

1.3 Diabetes

We have the same general picture for diabetes.

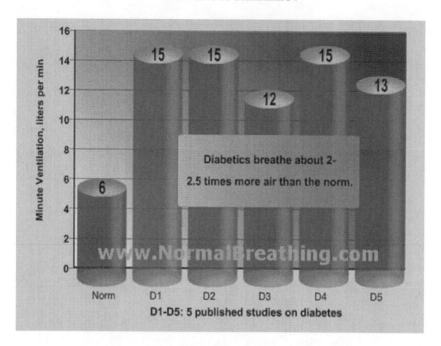

Table. Breathing rates in diabetics.

*One row corresponds to one medical study/publication

Minute ventilation rates in diabetics			
Condition	Minute ventilation	Number of people	References
Normal breathing	6 L/min	-	Medical textbooks
Healthy Subjects	6-7 L/min	>400	Results of 14 studies
Diabetes	12-17 L/min	26	Bottini et al, 2003
Diabetes	15 (±2) L/min	45	Tantucci et al, 2001
Diabetes	12 (±2) L/min	8	Mancini et al, 1999
Diabetes	10-20 L/min	28	Tantucci et al, 1997
Diabetes	13 (±2) L/min	20	Tantucci et al, 1996

References (in the same order)

18

Bottini P, Dottorini ML, M. Cordoni MC, Casucci G, Tantucci C, Sleep-disordered breathing in nonobese diabetic subjects with autonomic neuropathy, Eur Respir J 2003; 22: p. 654–660.

Tantucci C, Bottini P, Fiorani C, Dottorini ML, Santeusanio F, Provinciali L, Sorbini CA, Casucci G, Cerebrovascular reactivity and hypercapnic respiratory drive in diabetic autonomic neuropathy, J Appl Physiol 2001, 90: p. 889–896.

Mancini M, Filippelli M, Seghieri G, Iandelli I, Innocenti F, Duranti R, Scano G, Respiratory Muscle Function and Hypoxic Ventilatory Control in Patients With Type I Diabetes, Chest 1999; 115; p.1553-1562.

Tantucci C, Scionti L, Bottini P, Dottorini ML, Puxeddu E, Casucci G, Sorbini CA, Influence of autonomic neuropathy of different severities on the hypercapnic drive to breathing in diabetic patients, Chest. 1997 Jul; 112(1): p. 145-153.

Tantucci C, Bottini P, Dottorini ML, Puxeddu E, Casucci G, Scionti L, Sorbini CA, Ventilatory response to exercise in diabetic subjects with autonomic neuropathy, J Appl Physiol 1996, 81(5): p.1978–1986.

1.4 Other chronic diseases and disorders

The following studies also show heavy breathing in sick people with cancer, COPD, liver cirrhosis, cystic fibrosis, epilepsy, panic disorder, bipolar disorder, etc.

Table. Minute ventilation in patients with other chronic conditions.

*One row corresponds to one medical study/publication

Condition	Minute ventilation	Number of people	References
Normal breathing	6 L/min	-	Medical textbooks
Healthy Subjects	6-7 L/min	>400	Results of 14 studies
Pulm hypertension	12 (±2) L/min	11	D'Alonzo et al, 1987
Cancer	12 (±2) L/min	40	Travers et al, 2008
COPD	14 (±2) L/min	12	Palange et al, 2001
COPD	12 (±2) L/min	10	Sinderby et al, 2001
COPD	14 L/min	3	Stulbarg et al, 2001
Sleep apnea	15 (±3) L/min	20	Radwan et al, 2001
Liver cirrhosis	11-18 L/min	24	Epstein et al, 1998
Hyperthyroidism	15 (±1) L/min	42	Kahaly, 1998
Cystic fibrosis	15 L/min	15	Fauroux et al, 2006
Cystic fibrosis	10 L/min	11	Browning et al, 1990
Cystic fibrosis*	10 L/min	10	Ward et al, 1999
CF and diabetes*	10 L/min	7	Ward et al, 1999
Cystic fibrosis	16 L/min	7	Dodd et al, 2006
Cystic fibrosis	18 L/min	9	McKone et al, 2005
Cystic fibrosis*	13 (±2) L/min	10	Bell et al, 1996
Cystic fibrosis	11-14 L/min	6	Tepper et al, 1983
Epilepsy	13 L/min	12	Esquivel et al, 1991
CHV	13 (±2) L/min	134	Han et al, 1997
Panic disorder	12 (±5) L/min	12	Pain et al, 1991
Bipolar disorder	11 (±2) L/min	16	MacKinnon et al, 2007
Dystrophia myotonica	16 (±4) L/min	12	Clague et al, 1994

There are many more published studies obtaining the same results: **Sick people breathe too much.** In fact, all of the studies which I have found demonstrated the same conclusion (100% prevalence of overbreathing in the sick). Why is the minute ventilation test frequently done on heart patients rather than, for example, people with cancer? Heart patients often perform a "stress test" and minute ventilation is a normal parameter to be found and recorded during this test. Similarly, asthma and COPD patients routinely perform respiratory tests which are later published in medical journals. Hopefully, more awareness about the importance of normal breathing will result in more respiratory tests in relation to patients with cancer, GI problems, obesity, immune disorders and other chronic conditions.

References (in the same order)

D'Alonzo GE, Gianotti LA, Pohil RL, Reagle RR, DuRee SL, Fuentes F, Dantzker DR, Comparison of progressive exercise performance of normal subjects and patients with primary pulmonary hypertension, Chest 1987 Jul; 92(1): p.57-62.

Travers J, Dudgeon DJ, Amjadi K, McBride I, Dillon K, Laveneziana P, Ofir D, Webb KA, O'Donnell DE, Mechanisms of exertional dyspnea in patients with cancer, J Appl Physiol 2008 Jan; 104(1): p.57-66.

Palange P, Valli G, Onorati P, Antonucci R, Paoletti P, Rosato A, Manfredi F, Serra P, Effect of heliox on lung dynamic hyperinflation, dyspnea, and exercise endurance capacity in COPD patients, J Appl Physiol. 2004 Nov; 97(5): p.1637-1642.

Sinderby C, Spahija J, Beck J, Kaminski D, Yan S, Comtois N, Sliwinski P, Diaphragm activation during exercise in chronic obstructive pulmonary disease, Am J Respir Crit Care Med 2001 Jun; 163(7): 1637-1641.

Stulbarg MS, Winn WR, Kellett LE, Bilateral Carotid Body Resection for the Relief of Dyspnea in Severe Chronic Obstructive Pulmonary Disease, Chest 1989; 95 (5): p.1123-1128.

Radwan L, Maszczyk Z, Koziorowski A, Koziej M, Cieslicki J, Sliwinski P, Zielinski J, Control of breathing in obstructive sleep apnoea and in patients with the overlap syndrome, Eur Respir J. 1995 Apr; 8(4): p.542-545.

Epstein SK, Zilberberg MD; Facoby C, Ciubotaru RL, Kaplan LM, Response to symptom-limited exercise in patients with the hepatopulmonary syndrome, Chest 1998; 114; p. 736-741.

Kahaly GJ, Nieswandt J, Wagner S, Schlegel J, Mohr-Kahaly S, Hommel G, Ineffective cardiorespiratory function in hyperthyroidism, J Clin Endocrinol Metab 1998 Nov; 83(11): p. 4075-4078.

Bell SC, Saunders MJ, Elborn JS, Shale DJ, Resting energy expenditure and oxygen cost of breathing in patients with cystic fibrosis, Thorax 1996 Feb; 51(2): 126-131.

Tepper RS, Skatrud B, Dempsey JA, Ventilation and oxygenation changes during sleep in cystic fibrosis, Chest 1983; 84; p. 388-393.

Esquivel E, Chaussain M, Plouin P, Ponsot G, Arthuis M, Physical exercise and voluntary hyperventilation in childhood absence epilepsy, Electroencephalogr Clin Neurophysiol 1991 Aug; 79(2): p. 127-132.

Han JN, Stegen K, Simkens K, Cauberghs M, Schepers R, Van den Bergh O, Clément J, Van de Woestijne KP, Unsteadiness of breathing in patients with hyperventilation syndrome and anxiety disorders, Eur Respir J 1997; 10: p. 167–176.

Pain MC, Biddle N, Tiller JW, Panic disorder, the ventilatory response to carbon dioxide and respiratory variables, Psychosom Med 1988 Sep-Oct; 50(5): p. 541-548.

MacKinnon DF, Craighead B, Hoehn-Saric R, Carbon dioxide provocation of anxiety and respiratory response in bipolar disorder, J Affect Disord 2007 Apr; 99(1-3): p.45-49.

Clague JE, Carter J, Coakley J, Edwards RH, Calverley PM, Respiratory effort perception at rest and during carbon dioxide rebreathing in patients with dystrophia myotonica, Thorax 1994 Mar; 49(3): p.240-244.

2. Parameters of normal breathing

2.1 Physiological norms

Normal breathing is strictly nasal (in and out), mainly diaphragmatic (i.e., abdominal), slow (in frequency) and imperceptible (no feelings or sensation about one's own breathing at rest; see the explanation below). The physiological norm for minute ventilation at rest is 6 litres of air per minute for a 70 kg man (see references for textbooks below: Guyton, 1984; Ganong, 1995; Straub, 1998; Castro, 2000; etc.). These medical textbooks also provide the following parameters of normal breathing:
- normal tidal volume (air volume breathed in during a single breath): 500 ml;
- normal breathing frequency: 12 breaths per minute;
- normal inspiration: about 2 seconds;
- normal exhalation is 2-3 seconds.

The following graph represents the normal breathing pattern at rest or the dynamic of the volume of the lungs as a function of time:

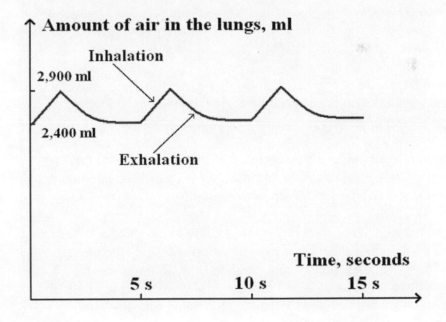

23

If a person with normal breathing is asked about their breathing sensations, they will testify that they do not feel their breathing. Why is this so? Normal tidal volume is only 500 ml or about 0.6 g of air, which is inhaled during one inspiration. Hence, normal breathing is slow in frequency and very small in amplitude. Sick people breathe deeper and faster. They often feel movements of air in the nose, chest movements, and other effects related to their deep and noisy breathing. Their deep breathing reduces body oxygenation and creates tissue hypoxia due to hypocapnic (low in CO_2) constriction of blood vessels and the suppressed Bohr effect discussed later.

2.2 Other parameters of normal breathing

"If a person breath-holds after a normal exhalation, it takes about 40 seconds before breathing commences" (McArdle et al, 2000). This indicates normal oxygenation of tissues.

The current medical norm for CO_2 content in the alveoli of the lungs and the arterial blood is 40 mm Hg CO_2. This number was established about a century ago by the famous British physiologists Charles G. Douglas and John S. Haldane from Oxford University. Their results were published in 1909 in the article "The regulation of normal breathing" by the Journal of Physiology (Douglas & Haldane, 1909).

Normal breathing is regular, invisible (no chest or belly movements), and inaudible (no panting, no wheezing, no sighing, no yawning, no sneezing, no coughing, no deep inhalations or exhalations).

In order to define one's breathing pattern, measure your body oxygenation or breath holding time after your usual exhalation, but only until the first sign of stress or discomfort.

The person with normal breathing is going to have about a 40 second breath holding time (or body oxygenation index). In the case of chronic over-breathing, breath holding time becomes shorter indicating reduced body oxygen stores. We are going to consider medical studies devoted to this breath holding time test later.

24

References: Medical and physiological textbooks

Ganong WF, Review of medical physiology, 15-th ed., 1995, Prentice Hall Int., London.

Guyton AC, Physiology of the human body, 6-th ed., 1984, Suanders College Publ., Philadelphia. McArdle W.D., Katch F.I., Katch V.L., Essentials of exercise physiology (2-nd edition); Lippincott,

Williams and Wilkins, London 2000.

Straub NC, Section V, The Respiratory System, in Physiology, eds. RM Berne & MN Levy, 4-th edition, Mosby, St. Louis, 1998.

Summary of values useful in pulmonary physiology: man. Section: Respiration and Circulation, ed. by P.L. Altman & D.S. Dittmer, 1971, Bethesda, Maryland (Federation of American Societies for Experimental Biology).

2.3 Myths about breathing and body oxygenation (prevalence: over 90%)

Myth #1. My breathing is OK and I know how to breathe.

Less than 10% of people have normal breathing parameters and body oxygen stores these days. We are going to consider 24 medical and physiological respiratory studies done on ordinary subjects during last 80 years. It is a fact that the medical norm established about a century ago is not a norm anymore. Modern people breathe about 2 times more air than we did 100 years ago. Hyperventilation results in tissue hypoxia and many other biochemical abnormalities (read Myth #3 below). Your breathing is normal, if and only if you have normal body oxygenation. How can you check it? You should be able to easily hold your breath for at least 40 seconds after your usual exhalation and with no stress at the end of the test. This test is described in detail later.

Myth #2. More breathing (deeper and/or greater volume) means better body oxygenation.

There is zero scientific evidence about this deep breathing myth, but hundreds of published studies have clearly shown that hyperventilation (or breathing more than the tiny medical norm) reduces oxygen supply to the brain, heart, liver, kidneys, and all other vital organs. Nevertheless, on TV, radio, and in everyday life situations, people who have little knowledge of physiology say, "Take a deep breath, get more oxygen", or "Breathe deeper for better oxygenation", etc.

Myth #3. Breathing is regulated by want for oxygen.

If you open any medical or physiological textbook with the description of the control of respiration, you will find that in normal conditions, breathing is regulated by the CO_2 concentration in the arterial blood and the brain. Whatever we do (sit, walk, eat, run, sleep, etc.), CO_2 concentration is kept within a narrow range (0.1% accuracy) by the breathing centre located in the medulla oblongata of the brain.

Myth #4. CO_2 is a poisonous or toxic gas and a waste product to get rid off.

When a healthy person tries to hyperventilate or is forced to breathe deeply and fast, he experiences "hypocapnia" (CO_2 deficiency) in the blood and other fluids, tissues, and cells. The immediate effects are:

- **constriction of blood vessels** (CO_2 is a powerful vasodilator) and reduced blood and oxygen supply to the brain, heart and all other vital organs (This is the reason why it is so easy to faint or pass out after 2-3 minutes of forceful hyperventilation. Horses and dogs died in 15-20 minutes, when they were forced to hyperventilate by a suction and exhaust pump)

- **the suppressed Bohr effect** or diminished release of oxygen by the blood in the tissues due to the same hypocapnia. Apart from these phenomena, there are many other vital functions of CO_2 in the human body. Meanwhile, reduced tissue oxygenation is sufficient to promote cancer, heart disease, diabetes and many other chronic conditions in case of overbreathing.

Myth #5. When a person is healthy, they can feel how they breathe.

If people with normal breathing are asked what they feel about their breathing, they will say that they feel nothing at all (as if they are barely breathing). "The perfect man breathes as if he is not breathing" Lao-Tzu, circa 4th century BC. Indeed, if you have any healthy people around you and observe their breathing for 20-30 seconds, you will see and hear nothing. The medical norm for breathing (6 L/min) is tiny.

Myth #6. Sick people notice when their breathing becomes abnormal.

100% prevalence of hyperventilation at rest for the sick people at rest is confirmed by over 20 published western studies on heart disease, cancer, asthma, COPD, diabetes, cystic fibrosis, epilepsy, panic attacks, chronic fatigue, and many other conditions. These sick patients breathe about 2-3 times more than the norm, and usually do not complain or even notice that their breathing is heavy or too deep. Why? Because air is weightless and the main breathing muscles (diaphragm and chest) are very powerful: we can pump 25 times more air during maximum exercise (or about 150 litres of air in one minute), than we require for normal breathing at rest (only about 6 L/min). People may notice that their breathing is heavy during heart attacks, stroke, asthma attacks, or morning hyperventilation (between 4 and 7 am), when chronically sick people are most likely to die from acute episodes triggered by hyperventilation.

One may easily confirm that most their relatives, friends, and other people do believe in these myths. My observations (about 90%

Dr. Artour Rakhimov

prevalence of these myths among the general population) are based on conversations with thousands of people.

2.4 Do modern healthy people also overbreathe?

We see that, according to these14 recent medical studies, healthy people still breathe little.

Table. Minute ventilation at rest in healthy subjects

Condition	Minute ventilation	N. of subjects	References
Normal breathing	6 L/min	-	Medical textbooks
Healthy subjects	7.7 ± 0.3 L/min	19	Douglas et al, 1982
Healthy males	8.4 ± 1.3 L/min	10	Burki, 1984
Healthy males	6.3 L/min	10	Smits et al, 1987
Healthy males	6.1±1.4 L/min	6	Fuller et al, 1987
Healthy subjects	6.1± 0.9 L/min	9	Tanaka et al, 1988
Healthy students	7.0 ± 1.0 L/min	10	Turley et al, 1993
Healthy subjects	6.6 ± 0.6 L/min	10	Bengtsson et al, 1994
Healthy subjects	7.0±1.2 L/min	12	Sherman et al, 1996
Healthy subjects	7.0±1.2 L/min	10	Bell et al, 1996
Healthy subjects	6 ± 1 L/min	7	Parreira et al, 1997
Healthy subjects	7.0 ± 1.1 L/min	14	Mancini et al, 1999
Healthy subjects	6.6 ± 1.1 L/min	40	Pinna et al, 2006
Healthy subjects	6.7 ± 0.5 L/min	17	Pathak et al, 2006
Healthy subjects	6.7 ± 0.3 L/min	14	Gujic et al, 2007

References for the Table (in the same order)

Douglas NJ, White DP, Pickett CK, Weil JV, Zwillich CW, Respiration during sleep in normal man, Thorax. 1982 Nov; 37(11): p.840-844.

Burki NK, Ventilatory effects of doxapram in conscious human subjects, Chest 1984 May; 85(5): p.600-604.

Smits P, Schouten J, Thien T, Respiratory stimulant effects of adenosine in man after caffeine and enprofylline, Br J Clin Pharmacol. 1987 Dec; 24(6): p.816-819.

Fuller RW, Maxwell DL, Conradson TB, Dixon CM, Barnes PJ, Circulatory and respiratory effects of infused adenosine in conscious man, Br J Clin Pharmacol 1987 Sep; 24(3): p.306-317.

Tanaka Y, Morikawa T, Honda Y, An assessment of nasal functions in control of breathing, J of Appl Physiol 1988, 65 (4); p.1520-1524.

Turley KR,McBride PJ, Wilmore LH, Resting metabolic rate measured after subjects spent the night at home vs at a clinic, Am J of Clin Nutr 1993, 58, p.141-144.

Bengtsson J, Bengtsson A, Stenqvist O, Bengtsson JP, Effects of hyperventilation on the inspiratory to end- tidal oxygen difference, British J of Anaesthesia 1994; 73: p. 140-144.

Sherman MS, Lang DM, Matityahu A, Campbell D, Theophylline improves measurements of respiratory muscle efficiency, Chest 1996 Dec; 110(6): p. 437-414.

Bell SC, Saunders MJ, Elborn JS, Shale DJ, Resting energy expenditure and oxygen cost of breathing in patients with cystic fibrosis, Thorax 1996 Feb; 51(2): 126-131.

Parreira VF, Delguste P, Jounieaux V, Aubert G, Dury M, Rodenstein DO, Effectiveness of controlled and spontaneous modes in nasal two-level positive pressure ventilation in awake and asleep normal subjects, Chest 1997 Nov 5; 112(5): p.1267-1277.

Mancini M, Filippelli M, Seghieri G, Iandelli I, Innocenti F, Duranti R, Scano G, Respiratory Muscle Function and Hypoxic Ventilatory Control in Patients With Type I Diabetes, Chest 1999; 115; p.1553-1562.

Pinna GD, Maestri R, La Rovere MT, Gobbi E, Fanfulla F, Effect of paced breathing on ventilatory and cardiovascular variability parameters during short-term investigations of autonomic function, Am J Physiol Heart Circ Physiol. 2006 Jan; 290(1): p.H424-433.

Pathak A, Velez-Roa S, Xhaët O, Najem B, van de Borne P, Dose-dependent effect of dobutamine on chemoreflex activity in healthy volunteers, Br J Clin Pharmacol. 2006 Sep; 62(3): p.272-279.

Gujic M, Houssière A, Xhaët O, Argacha JF, Denewet N, Noseda A, Jespers P, Melot C, Naeije R, van de Borne P, Does endothelin play a role in chemoreception during acute hypoxia in normal men? Chest. 2007 May; 131(5): p.1467-1472.

2.5 What about historical changes in breathing of ordinary people?

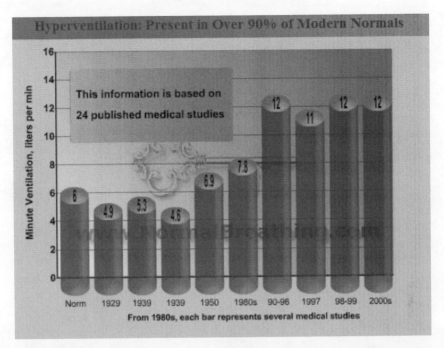

The table below represents results of 24 medical studies (from 1929 until 2007). It tells us that before WW2 breathing rates of ordinary people were even less than normal. During last 2 decades ordinary people breathe about 2 times more air than the medical norm.

Table. Historical changes in minute ventilation at rest for normal subjects

Condition	Minute ventilation	Age	N. of subjects	References
Healthy Subjects	6-7 L/min	-	>400	Results of 14 studies
Normal breathing	6	-	-	Medical textbooks
Normal subjects	4.9	-	5	Griffith et al, 1929
Normal males	5.3±0.1	27-43	46	Shock et al, 1939
Normal females	4.6±0.1	27-43	40	Shock et al, 1939
Normal subjects	6.9±0.9	-	100	Matheson et al, 1950
Normal subjects	9.1±4.5	31±7	11	Kassabian et al, 1982
Normal subjects	8.1±2.1	42±14	11	D'Alonzo et al, 1987
Normal subjects	6.3±2.2	-	12	Pain et al, 1988
Normal males	13±3	40 (av.)	12	Clague et al, 1994
Normal subjects	9.2±2.5	34±7	13	Radwan et al, 1995
Normal subjects	15±4	28-34	12	Dahan et al, 1995
Normal subjects	12±4	55±10	43	Clark et al, 1995
Normal subjects	12±2	41±2	10	Tantucci et al, 1996
Normal subjects*	11±3	53±11	24	Clark et al, 1997

Condition	Minute ventilation	Age	N. of subjects	Reference
Normal subjects	8.1±0.4	34±2	63	Meessen et al, 1997
Normal females	9.9	20-28	23	Han et al, 1997
Normal males	15	20-28	47	Han et al, 1997
Normal females	10	29-60	42	Han et al, 1997
Normal males	11	29-62	42	Han et al, 1997
Normal subjects	13±3	36±6	10	Tantucci et al, 1997
Normal subjects	12±1	65±2	10	Epstein et al, 1996
Normal subjects	12±1	12-69	20	Bowler et al, 1998
Normal subjects	10±6	39±4	20	DeLorey et al, 1999
Normal seniors	12±4	70±3	14	DeLorey et al, 1999
Normal elderly*	14±3	88±2	11	DeLorey et al, 1999
Normal subjects	17±1	41±2	15	Tantucci et al, 2001
Normal subjects	10±0.5	-	10	Bell et al, 2005
Normal subjects	8.5±1.2	30±8	69	Narkiewicz, 2006
Normal females	10±0.4	-	11	Ahuja et al, 2007
Normal subjects	12±2	62±2	20	Travers et al, 2008

* When the average weight of the subjects was significantly different from 70 kg, minute ventilation was adjusted to the normal weight (70 kg) value.

Note that the results are inconsistent since there is no strict definition for "normal" or "control" subjects in medical research. Consider a medical study with a group of asthmatics. If the organizers of the study want to see the effects of some medication or treatment on these asthmatics, the researchers may also select a group of control subjects for comparison. These "control" subjects must be either asthma-free or they must be free from any serious health problems and symptoms.

References for the Table (in the same order)

Griffith FR, Pucher GW, Brownell KA, Klein JD, Carmer ME, Studies in human physiology. IV. Vital capacity, respiratory rate and volume, and composition of the expired air. Am. J. Physiol 1929, vol. 89, p. 555.

Shock NW, Soley MH, Average Values for Basal Respiratory Functions in Adolescents and Adults, J. Nutrition, 1939, 18, p. 143.

Matheson HW, Gray JS, Ventilatory function tests. III Resting ventilation, metabolism, and derived measures, J Clin Invest 1950 June; 29(6): p. 688–692.

Kassabian J, Miller KD, Lavietes MH, Respiratory center output and ventilatory timing in patients with acute airway (asthma) and alveolar (pneumonia) disease, Chest 1982 May; 81(5): p.536-543.

D'Alonzo GE, Gianotti LA, Pohil RL, Reagle RR, DuRee SL, Fuentes F, Dantzker DR, Comparison of progressive exercise performance of normal subjects and patients with primary pulmonary hypertension, Chest 1987 Jul; 92(1): p.57-62.

Pain MC, Biddle N, Tiller JW, Panic disorder, the ventilatory response to carbon dioxide and respiratory variables, Psychosom Med 1988 Sep-Oct; 50(5): p. 541-548.

Clague JE, Carter J, Coakley J, Edwards RH, Calverley PM, Respiratory effort perception at rest and during carbon dioxide rebreathing in patients with dystrophia myotonica, Thorax 1994 Mar; 49(3): p.240-244.

Radwan L, Maszczyk Z, Koziorowski A, Koziej M, Cieslicki J, Sliwinski P, Zielinski J, Control of breathing in obstructive sleep apnoea and in patients with the overlap syndrome, Eur Respir J. 1995 Apr; 8(4): p.542-545.

Dahan A, van den Elsen MJ, Berkenbosch A, DeGoede J, Olievier IC, van Kleef JW, Halothane affects ventilatory afterdischarge in humans, Br J Anaesth 1995 May; 74(5): p.544-548.

Clark AL, Chua TP, Coats AJ, Anatomical dead space, ventilatory pattern, and exercise capacity in chronic heart failure, Br Heart J 1995 Oct; 74(4): p. 377-380.

Tantucci C, Bottini P, Dottorini ML, Puxeddu E, Casucci G, Scionti L, Sorbini CA, Ventilatory response to exercise in diabetic subjects with autonomic neuropathy, J Appl Physiol 1996, 81(5): p.1978–1986.

Clark AL, Volterrani M, Swan JW, Coats AJS, The increased ventilatory response to exercise in chronic heart failure: relation to pulmonary pathology, Heart 1997; 77: p.138-146.

Meessen NE, van der Grinten CP, Luijendijk SC, Folgering HT, Breathing pattern during bronchial challenge in humans, Eur Respir J 1997 May; 10(5): p.1059-1063.

Han JN, Stegen K, Simkens K, Cauberghs M, Schepers R, Van den Bergh O, Clément J, Van de Woestijne KP, Unsteadiness of breathing in patients with hyperventilation syndrome and anxiety disorders, Eur Respir J 1997; 10: p. 167–176.

Tantucci C, Scionti L, Bottini P, Dottorini ML, Puxeddu E, Casucci G, Sorbini CA, Influence of autonomic neuropathy of different severities on the hypercapnic drive to breathing in diabetic patients, Chest. 1997 Jul; 112(1): 145-153.

Epstein SK, Zilberberg MD; Facoby C, Ciubotaru RL, Kaplan LM, Response to symptom-limited exercise in patients with the hepatopulmonary syndrome, Chest 1998; 114; p. 736-741.

Bowler SD, Green A, Mitchell CA, Buteyko breathing techniques in asthma: a blinded randomised controlled trial, Med J of Australia 1998; 169: p. 575-578.

DeLorey DS, Babb TG, Progressive mechanical ventilatory constraints with aging, Am J Respir Crit Care Med 1999 Jul; 160(1): p.169-177.

Tantucci C, Bottini P, Fiorani C, Dottorini ML, Santeusanio F, Provinciali L, Sorbini CA, Casucci G, Cerebrovascular reactivity and hypercapnic respiratory drive in diabetic autonomic neuropathy, J Appl Physiol 2001, 90: p. 889–896.

Bell HJ, Feenstra W, Duffin J, The initial phase of exercise hyperpnoea in humans is depressed during a cognitive task, Experimental Physiology 2005 May; 90(3): p.357-365.

Narkiewicz K, van de Borne P, Montano N, Hering D, Kara T, Somers VK, Sympathetic neural outflow and chemoreflex sensitivity are related to spontaneous breathing rate in normal men, Hypertension 2006 Jan; 47(1): p.51-55.

Ahuja D, Mateika JH, Diamond MP, Badr MS, Ventilatory sensitivity to carbon dioxide before and after episodic hypoxia in women treated with testosterone, J Appl Physiol. 2007 May; 102(5): p.1832-1838.

Travers J, Dudgeon DJ, Amjadi K, McBride I, Dillon K, Laveneziana P, Ofir D, Webb KA, O'Donnell DE, Mechanisms of exertional dyspnea in patients with cancer, J Appl Physiol 2008 Jan; 104(1): p.57-66.

3. Effects of overbreathing (hyperventilation)

3.1 Hypocapnia (or CO2 deficiency in the blood and cells)

When a person starts to over-breathe or hyperventilate (breathe more air per minute), blood oxygenation in the lungs has a negligible increase. Why? During normal breathing haemoglobin cells of the arterial blood have 98-99% O2 saturation. Hence, more breathing cannot increase blood oxygenation to any significant degree.

If a healthy person starts to breathe more or deeper, what are the other effects?
- More carbon dioxide is removed from the lungs with each breath and therefore the level of CO2 in the lungs immediately decreases
- In 1-2 minutes, the CO2 level falls below the normal levels in all the blood due to its circulation
- In 3-5 minutes, due to CO2 diffusion, most cells of the body (including vital organs and muscles) experience lowered CO2 concentrations
- In 15-20 minutes, the CO2 level in the brain is below the norm due to a slower diffusion rate.

3.2 Vasoconstriction

As independent physiological studies found, hypocapnia (low CO2 concentration in the arterial blood) decreased perfusion of the following organs:
- brain (Fortune et al, 1995; Karlsson et al, 1994; Liem et al, 1995; Macey et al, 2007; Santiago & Edelman, 1986; Starling & Evans, 1968; Tsuda et al, 1987)
- heart (Coetzee et al, 1984; Foëx et al, 1979; Karlsson et al, 1994; Okazaki et al, 1991; Okazaki et al, 1992; Wexels et al, 1985)
- liver (Dutton et al, 1976; Fujita et al, 1989; Hughes et al, 1979; Okazaki, 1989)

- kidneys (Karlsson et al, 1994; Okazaki, 1989)
- spleen (Karlsson et al, 1994)
- colon (Gilmour et al, 1980).

Some abstracts of these studies are provided at the bottom of this page.

What is the physiological mechanism of the reduced blood flow to vital organs? CO_2 is a dilator of blood vessels (arteries and arterioles). Arteries and arterioles have their own tiny smooth muscles that can constrict or dilate depending on CO_2 concentrations. When we breathe more, CO_2 level in the arterial blood decreases, blood vessels constrict and vital organs (like the brain, heart, kidneys, liver, stomach, spleen, colon, etc.) get less blood supply.

Are there any related systemic effects? The state of these blood vessels (arteries and arterioles) defines the total resistance to the systemic blood flow in the human body. Hence, hypocapnia increases the strain on the heart. Hence, breathing directly participates in regulation of the heart rate. The father of cardiorespiratory physiology, Yale University Professor Yandell Henderson (1873-1944), investigated this effect about a century ago.

Among his numerous physiological studies, he performed experiments with anaesthetized dogs on mechanical ventilation. The results were described in his publication "*Acapnia and shock. - I. Carbon dioxide as a factor in the regulation of the heart rate*". In this article, published in 1908 in the American Journal of Physiology, he wrote, "... *we were enabled to regulate the heart to any desired rate from 40 or fewer up to 200 or more beats per minute. The method was very simple. It depended on the manipulation of the hand bellows with which artificial respiration was administered... As the pulmonary ventilation increased or diminished the heart rate was correspondingly accelerated or retarded*" (p.127, Henderson, 1908).

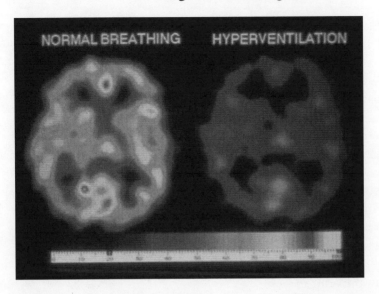

Other medical observations

Imagine that a person at rest starts to hyperventilate or breathe very heavy and fast. What would happen? The person would feel dizzy and could faint or pass out. Why? It cannot be due to too much oxygen, since their blood is almost fully saturated with O2 with very shallow (or normal) breathing at rest. This scan shows brain oxygenation in two conditions: normal breathing and after 1 minute of hyperventilation. The red color represents the most O2, dark blue the least. Brain oxygenation for overbreathing is reduced by 40% (Litchfield, 2003).

This result is quoted in many medical textbooks (e.g., Starling & Evans, 1968) since the effect is well documented and has been confirmed by dozens of professional experiments. According to the Handbook of Physiology (Santiago & Edelman, 1986), cerebral blood flow decreases 2% for every mm Hg decrease in CO2 pressure. Why?

Be observant. When you get a small bleeding cut or a wound, deliberately hyperventilate and see if that can help stop the bleeding. It should happen. As an alternative, perform comfortable breath holding and breathe less and accumulate CO2. What would happen with your bleeding? (It should increase.) Now you know what to do after dental surgeries, brain traumas, and other accidents involving bleeding. It is natural for humans and other animals to breathe heavily in such conditions. Hence, hyperventilation can be life saving in cases of severe bleeding.

Why did Nature provide us with this physiological reaction: vasoconstriction due to hyperventilation? Breathing is closely connected with blood flow to all vital organs, sensitivity of the immune system, permeability of cellular membranes, and many other functions. As soon as vital organs (the brain, heart, stomach, kidneys, liver, etc.) are under stress (chemical, viral, bacteriological, etc.), or inflammation, or injury, the breathing gets heavier.

That helps to prevent:
- excessive bleeding (as in cases of open injuries, cuts, bruises, etc.)
- quick spread of bacterial and viral infections
- excessive amounts of toxic products in the blood from injured, infected, or polluted tissues
- damage to vital cleansing organs (e.g., liver and kidneys) due to their possible toxic overload.

All these preventive effects can save the life of the organism in the short run. At the same time, it is not normal to be in a state of stress (chronic hyperventilation) all the time. Our breathing, if there is no emergency, should be normal.

References

Coetzee A, Holland D, Foëx P, Ryder A, Jones L, The effect of hypocapnia on coronary blood flow and myocardial function in the dog, Anesthesia and Analgesia 1984 Nov; 63(11): p. 991-997.

Dutton R, Levitzky M, Berkman R, Carbon dioxide and liver blood flow, Bull Eur Physiopathol Respir. 1976 Mar-Apr; 12(2): p. 265-273.

Gilmour DG, Douglas IH, Aitkenhead AR, Hothersall AP, Horton PW, Ledingham IM, Colon blood flow in the dog: effects of changes in arterial carbon dioxide tension, Cardiovasc Res 1980 Jan; 14(1): 11-20.

Foëx P, Ryder WA, Effect of CO2 on the systemic and coronary circulations and on coronary sinus blood gas tensions, Bull Eur Physiopathol Respir 1979 Jul-Aug; 15(4): p.625-638.

Fortune JB, Feustel PJ, deLuna C, Graca L, Hasselbarth J, Kupinski AM, Cerebral blood flow and blood volume in response to O2 and CO2 changes in normal humans, J Trauma. 1995 Sep; 39(3): p. 463-471. Fujita Y, Sakai T, Ohsumi A, Takaori M, Effects of hypocapnia and hypercapnia on splanchnic circulation and hepatic function in the beagle, Anesthesia and Analgesia 1989 Aug; 69(2): p. 152-157.

Hashimoto K, Okazaki K, Okutsu Y, The effects of hypocapnia and hypercapnia on tissue surface PO2 in hemorrhaged dogs [Article in Japanese], Masui 1989 Oct; 38(10): p. 1271-1274.

Henderson Y, Acapnia and shock. - I. Carbon dioxide as a factor in the regulation of the heart rate, American Journal of Physiology 1908, 21: p. 126-156.

Hughes RL, Mathie RT, Fitch W, Campbell D, Liver blood flow and oxygen consumption during hypocapnia and IPPV in the greyhound, J Appl Physiol. 1979 Aug; 47(2): p. 290-295.

Karlsson T, Stjernström EL, Stjernström H, Norlén K, Wiklund L, Central and regional blood flow during hyperventilation. An experimental study in the pig, Acta Anaesthesiol Scand. 1994 Feb; 38(2): p.180-186. Liem KD, Kollée LA, Hopman JC, De Haan AF, Oeseburg B, The influence of arterial carbon dioxide on cerebral oxygenation and haemodynamics during ECMO in normoxaemic and hypoxaemic piglets, Acta Anaesthesiol Scand Suppl. 1995; 107: p.157-164.

Litchfield PM, A brief overview of the chemistry of respiration and the breathing heart wave, California Biofeedback, 2003 Spring, 19(1).

Macey PM, Woo MA, Harper RM, Hyperoxic brain effects are normalized by addition of CO2, PLoS Med. 2007 May; 4(5): p. e173.

McArdle WD, Katch FI, Katch VL, Essentials of exercise physiology (2-nd edition); Lippincott, Williams and Wilkins, London 2000.

Okazaki K, Okutsu Y, Fukunaga A, Effect of carbon dioxide (hypocapnia and hypercapnia) on tissue blood flow and oxygenation of liver, kidneys and skeletal muscle in the dog, Masui 1989 Apr, 38 (4): p. 457-464. Okazaki K, Hashimoto K, Okutsu Y, Okumura F, Effect of arterial carbon dioxide tension on regional myocardial tissue oxygen tension in the dog [Article in Japanese], Masui 1991 Nov; 40(11): p. 1620-1624. Okazaki K, Hashimoto K, Okutsu Y, Okumura F, Effect of carbon dioxide (hypocapnia and hypercapnia) on regional myocardial tissue oxygen tension in dogs with coronary stenosis [Article in Japanese], Masui 1992 Feb; 41(2): p. 221-224.

Santiago TV & Edelman NH, Brain blood flow and control of breathing, in Handbook of Physiology, Section 3: The respiratory system, vol. II, ed. by AP Fishman. American Physiological Society, Betheda, Maryland, 1986, p. 163-179.

Starling E & Lovatt EC, Principles of human physiology, 14-th ed., 1968, Lea & Febiger, Philadelphia. Tsuda Y, Kimura K, Yoneda S, Hartmann A, Etani H, Hashikawa K, Kamada T, Effect of hypocapnia on cerebral oxygen metabolism and blood flow in ischemic cerebrovascular disorders, Eur Neurol. 1987; 27(3): p.155-163.

Wexels JC, Myhre ES, Mjøs OD, Effects of carbon dioxide and pH on myocardial blood-flow and metabolism in the dog, Clin Physiol. 1985 Dec; 5(6): p.575-588.

3.3 Suppressed Bohr effect

Why do hemoglobin cells of the arterial blood release oxygen in the
tissues, not in the arteries, or arterioles, or veins? Why is more
oxygen released in those tissues of the human body that produce
more energy? These processes depend on local CO_2 content due to
the Bohr law (or Bohr effect). The effect was first described in 1904
by the Danish physiologist Christian Bohr (father of famous
physicist Niels Bohr). He stated that at higher CO_2 content in tissues
(more acidic environment), hemoglobin will bind to oxygen with
less affinity. Hence, those tissues that generate more CO_2 will get
more oxygen from the blood.

There are many modern professional investigations devoted to
various aspects of this effect (e.g., Braumann et al, 1982; Böning et
al, 1975; Bucci et al, 1985; Carter et al, 1985; diBella et al, 1986;
Dzhagarov et al, 1996; Grant et al, 1982; Grubb et al, 1979;
Gersonde et al, 1986; Hlastala & Woodson, 1983; Jensen, 2004;
Kister et al, 1988; Kobayashi et al, 1989; Lapennas, 1983; Matthew
et al, 1979; Meyer et al, 1978; Tyuma, 1984; Winslow et al, 1985).

Hyperventilation or reduced CO_2 tissue tension leads to hampered
oxygen release and reduced oxygen tension in tissues (Aarnoudse et
al, 1981; Monday & Tétreault, 1980; Gottstein et al, 1976). In order
to improve the release of oxygen by red blood cells, we require more
CO_2 in the cells and the whole body. Hence, we should learn how to
breathe less for better body oxygenation.

References

Aarnoudse JG, Oeseburg B, Kwant G, Zwart A, Zijlstra WG,
Huisjes HJ, Influence of variations in pH and PCO_2 on scalp tissue
oxygen tension and carotid arterial oxygen tension in the fetal lamb,
Biol Neonate 1981; 40(5-6): p. 252-263.

Braumann KM, Böning D, Trost F, Bohr effect and slope of the
oxygen dissociation curve after physical training, J Appl Physiol.
1982 Jun; 52(6): p. 1524-1529.

Böning D, Schwiegart U, Tibes U, Hemmer B, Influences of exercise and endurance training on the oxygen dissociation curve of blood under in vivo and in vitro conditions, Eur J Appl Physiol Occup Physiol. 1975; 34(1): p. 1-10.

Bucci E, Fronticelli C, Anion Bohr effect of human hemoglobin, Biochemistry. 1985 Jan 15; 24(2): p. 371-376.

Carter AM, Grønlund J, Contribution of the Bohr effect to the fall in fetal PO2 caused by maternal alkalosis, J Perinat Med. 1985; 13(4): p.185-191.

diBella G, Scandariato G, Suriano O, Rizzo A, Oxygen affinity and Bohr effect responses to 2,3- diphosphoglycerate in equine and human blood, Res Vet Sci. 1996 May; 60(3): p. 272-275.

Dzhagarov BM, Kruk NN, The alkaline Bohr effect: regulation ofthnded hemoglobin Hb(O2)3 [Article in Russian] Biofizika. 1996 May-Jun; 41(3): p. 606-612.

Gersonde K, Sick H, Overkamp M, Smith KM, Parish DW, Bohr effect in monomeric insect haemoglobins controlled by O2 off-rate and modulated by haem-rotational disorder, Eur J Biochem. 1986 Jun 2; 157(2): p. 393-404.

Grant BJ, Influence of Bohr-Haldane effect on steady-state gas exchange, J Appl Physiol. 1982 May; 52(5): p. 1330-1337.

Grubb B, Jones JH, Schmidt-Nielsen K, Avian cerebral blood flow: influence of the Bohr effect on oxygen supply, Am J Physiol. 1979 May; 236(5): p. H744-749.

Gottstein U, Zahn U, Held K, Gabriel FH, Textor T, Berghoff W, Effect of hyperventilation on cerebral blood flow and metabolism in man; continuous monitoring of arterio-cerebral venous glucose differences (author's transl) [Article in German], Klin Wochenschr. 1976 Apr 15; 54(8): p. 373-381.

Hlastala MP, Woodson RD, Bohr effect data for blood gas calculations, J Appl Physiol. 1983 Sep; 55(3): p. 1002-1007.

Jensen FB, Red blood cell pH, the Bohr effect, and other oxygenation-linked phenomena in blood O2 and CO2 transport, Acta Physiol Scand. 2004 Nov; 182(3): p. 215-227.

Kister J, Marden MC, Bohn B, Poyart C, Functional properties of hemoglobin in human red cells: II. Determination of the Bohr effect, Respir Physiol. 1988 Sep; 73(3): p. 363-378.

Kobayashi H, Pelster B, Piiper J, Scheid P, Significance of the Bohr effect for tissue oxygenation in a model with counter-current blood flow, Respir Physiol. 1989 Jun; 76(3): p. 277-288.

Lapennas GN, The magnitude of the Bohr coefficient: optimal for oxygen delivery, Respir Physiol. 1983 Nov; 54(2): p.161-172.

Matthew JB, Hanania GI, Gurd FR, Electrostatic effects in hemoglobin: Bohr effect and ionic strength dependence of individual groups, Biochemistry. 1979 May 15; 18(10): p.1928-1936.

Meyer M, Holle JP, Scheid P, Bohr effect induced by CO2 and fixed acid at various levels of O2 saturation in duck blood, Pflugers Arch. 1978 Sep 29; 376(3): p. 237-240.

Monday LA, Tétreault L, Hyperventilation and vertigo, Laryngoscope 1980 Jun; 90(6 Pt 1): p.1003-1010. Tyuma I, The Bohr effect and the Haldane effect in human hemoglobin, Jpn J Physiol. 1984; 34(2): p.205-216.

Winslow RM, Monge C, Winslow NJ, Gibson CG, Whittembury J, Normal whole blood Bohr effect in Peruvian natives of high altitude, Respir Physiol. 1985 Aug; 61(2): p. 197-208.

3.4 Less oxygen for cells

Summarizing these physiological laws and facts, we can conclude:

45

1. Hyperventilation cannot increase O2 content in the arterial blood to any significant degree (normal hemoglobin saturation is about 98%), but it reduces CO2 concentrations in all cells and the blood.

2. Hypocapnia (or CO2 deficiency) leads to constriction of blood vessels and that reduces blood supply to vital organs of the human body.

3. Hypocapnia (or CO2 deficiency) also leads to suppressed Bohr effect that causes further reduction in cellular oxygen delivery.

Hence, the more one breathes, the less oxygen is provided for vital organs.

The discussed effects of CO2-deficiency (hyperventilation) on blood circulation and oxygen transport are summarized on the graphs on the next page.

Normal gas exchanges

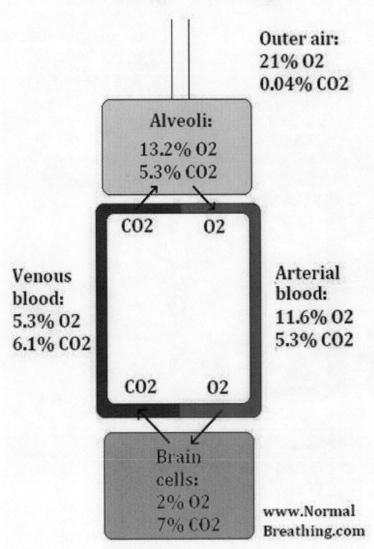

Effects of hyperventilation on circulation and normal gas exchange

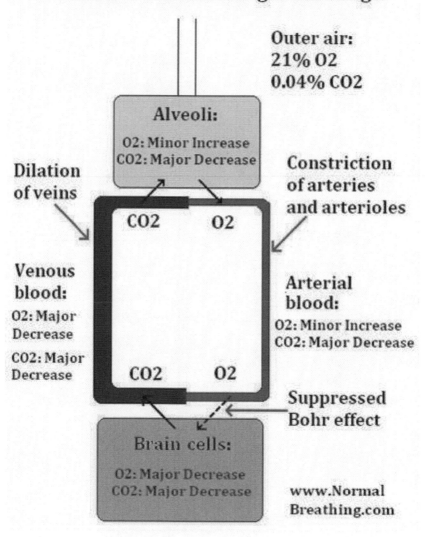

3.5 Other hypocapnia-related abnormalities

Among other effects of CO_2 deficiency are:
- abnormal excitability and irritability of nerve cells (e.g., Brown, 1953; Krnjevic, 1965; Balestrino & Somjen, 1988; Huttunen et al, 1999)
- irritable state of muscles (muscular tension) (Brown, 1953; Hudlicka, 1973)
- bronchoconstriction (or reduced diameter of airways causing wheezing and sensations of breathlessness and suffocation) (Sterling, 1968)
- abnormalities with ions in blood plasma and other bodily fluids (Carryer, 1947)
- innumerable abnormalities in chemical reactions involving synthesis of amino acids, lipids (fats), carbohydrates, hormones, messengers, cells of the immune system, etc.

Dr. Brown in his article "Physiological effects of hyperventilation" analyzed almost 300 professional studies and stated, "Studies designed to determine the effects produced by hyperventilation on nerve and muscle have been consistent in their finding on increased irritability" (Brown, 1953).

Other authors (Balestrino & Somjen, 1988; Huttunen et al, 1999) also concluded that increased CO_2 pressure generally reduces cortical excitability, while hyperventilation "leads to spontaneous and asynchronous firing of cortical neurons" (Huttunen et. al., 1999).

References

Balestrino M, Somjen GG, Concentration of carbon dioxide, interstitial pH and synaptic transmission in hippocampal formation of the rat, J Physiol 1988, 396: p. 247-266.

Brown EB, Physiological effects of hyperventilation, Physiol Reviews 1953 Oct, 33 (4): p. 445-471.

Carryer HM, Hyperventilation syndrome, Med Clin North Amer 1947, 31: p. 845.

Hudlicka O, Muscle blood flow, 1973, Swets&Zeitlinger, Amsterdam.

Huttunen J, Tolvanen H, Heinonen E, Voipio J, Wikstrom H, Ilmoniemi RJ, Hari R, Kaila K, Effects of voluntary hyperventilation on cortical sensory responses. Electroencephalographic and magnetoencephalographic studies, Exp Brain Res 1999, 125(3): p. 248-254.

Krnjevic K, Randic M and Siesjo B, Cortical CO2 tension and neuronal excitability, J of Physiol 1965, 176: p. 105-122.

Sterling GM, The mechanism of bronchoconstriction due to hypocapnia in man, Clin Sci 1968 Apr; 34(2): p. 277-285.

4. How to measure breathing and oxygenation

4.1 How to measure the CP (the index of oxygenation)

Measurement of the CP (control pause)

Sit down and rest for 5-7 minutes. Completely relax all your muscles, including the breathing muscles. This relaxation produces natural spontaneous exhalation (breathing out). Pinch your nose at the end of this exhalation and count your CP (breath holding time) in seconds. Keep the nose pinched until you experience the first desire to breathe, so that, after you release the fingers, you can resume your usual breathing (in the same way as you were breathing just before you started to hold your breath). Do not extend breath holding too long. You should not gasp for air or open your mouth afterwards. The test should be easy and must not cause you stress because it does not interfere with your breathing. Look at the diagram below: after the test you can comfortably breathe as before the test.

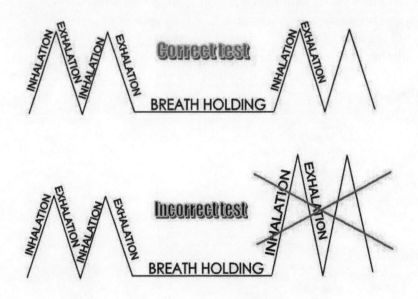

If you hold the breath for too long time (incorrect test), the first inhale will be large, deep and noisy, as on the graph above.

Now one can easily define their own health state at any moment of time. Since breathing and body oxygenation vary throughout the day, one's health parameters are usually worse during early morning hours and the MCP (morning Control Pause), according to Dr. Buteyko and his colleagues, is the main parameter that reflects personal health state. The MCP test is done as the first thing in the morning, while lying in bed.

It is important for future success, to write down your MCP every day. (The daily log is provided in Chapter 7 or can be downloaded from the website.)

The CP is the simplest and most accurate test of personal physical health for well over 97% of people. This physiological fact has been confirmed by many professional studies and experiences of thousands of formerly-sick people who recovered their health using breathing retraining.

Consider this graph with bars that summarize data from 9 independent medical publications. Each bar represents one physiological study with the title of the health condition studied and the number of patients (in brackets). The normal CP is about 40 seconds (the large blue bar). Shorter red bars corresponds to diseases states.

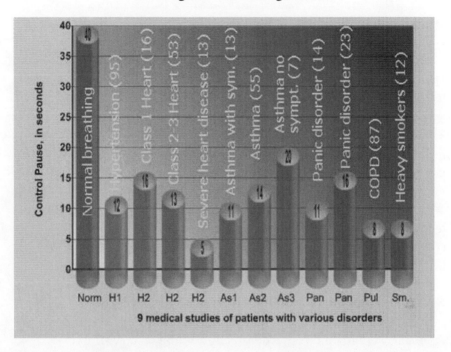

Note. For example, the first red bar on the left represents a medical study in which it was found that 95 patients with hypertension had, on average, 12 seconds of oxygen in the body instead of normal 40 seconds.

We can also easily observe here that the oxygenation index correlates well with severity of the severity of the disease for asthma and heart patients. For example, functional heart disease corresponds to about 5 seconds of oxygen in the body, moderate heart disease (class 2 US classification) to about 10 second CP, and light forms of heart disease to about 15 seconds. Similarly, asthmatics who experience symptoms have about 10 seconds of oxygen. In between attacks (or in stable conditions), asthmatics usually have about a 15 second CP. If they get up to a 20 second CP, they do not experience chest tightness, wheezing, blocked nose and other pathological effects.

In both cases, asthma and heart disease, patients generally do not require any medication and do not experience any negative symptoms, if their CP is above 20 seconds 24/7. The same observation has been found for bronchitis, sinusitis, chronic fatigue, eczema, epilepsy and many other disorders.

Hence, the first goal for most patients, in order to get more stable health and reasonable well-being is to have over 20 second CP 24/7.

The CP test not only defines oxygenation of the human body, it also tells us about your minute ventilation (or how much you breathe). If you have normal breathing, your CP should be about 40 seconds. If your CP is about 20 seconds, you breathe for 2 people. If your CP is 10 seconds, you breathe 4 times more than the norm. Hence, if you learn and practice some exercises that increase your body CO_2 content and try to breathe less 24/7, your CP will grow and your health will improve.

References for the graph (in the same order)

Ayman D, Goldshine AD, The breath-holding test. A simple standard stimulus of blood pressure, Archives of Intern Medicine 1939, 63; p. 899-906.

Friedman M, Studies concerning the aetiology and pathogenesis of neurocirculatory asthenia III. The cardiovascular manifestations of neurocirculatory asthenia, Am Heart J 1945; 30, 378-391.

Mirsky I A, Lipman E, Grinker R R, Breath-holding time in anxiety state, Federation proceedings 1946; 5: p.74.

Kohn RM & Cutcher B, Breath-holding time in the screening for rehabilitation potential of cardiac patients, Scand J Rehabil Med 1970; 2(2): p. 105-107.

Davidson JT, Whipp BJ, Wasserman K, Koyal SN, Lugliani R, Role of the carotid bodies in breath-holding, New England Journal of Medicine 1974 April 11; 290(15): p. 819-822.

Perez-Padilla R, Cervantes D, Chapela R, Selman M, Rating of breathlessness at rest during acute asthma: correlation with spirometry and usefulness of breath-holding time, Rev Invest Clin 1989 Jul-Sep; 41(3): p. 209-213.

Zandbergen J, Strahm M, Pols H, Griez EJ, Breath-holding in panic disorder, Compar Psychiatry 1992 Jan- Feb; 33(1): p. 47-51.

Gay SB, Sistrom C1L, Holder CA, Suratt PM, Breath-holding capability of adults. Implications for spiral computed tomography, fast-acquisition magnetic resonance imaging, and angiography, Invest Radiol 1994 Sep; 29(9): p. 848-851.

Asmundson GJ & Stein MB, Triggering the false suffocation alarm in panic disorder patients by using a voluntary breath-holding procedure, Am J Psychiatry 1994 Feb; 151(2): p. 264-266.

Taskar V, Clayton N, Atkins M, Shaheen Z, Stone P, Woodcock A, Breath-holding time in normal subjects, snorers, and sleep apnea patients, Chest 1995 Apr; 107(4): p. 959-962.

Marks B, Mitchell DG, Simelaro JP, Breath-holding in healthy and pulmonary-compromised populations: effects of hyperventilation and oxygen inspiration, J Magn Reson Imaging 1997 May-Jun; 7(3): p. 595-597. Nannini LJ, Zaietta GA, Guerrera AJ, Varela JA, Fernandez AM, Flores DM, Breath-holding test in subjects with near-fatal asthma. A new index for dyspnea perception, Respiratory Medicine 2007, 101; p.246–253.

4.2 MCP (morning CP): your main health parameter

Physiological, medical and epidemiological studies have clearly shown that people with severe forms of heart disease, asthma, COPD, epilepsy, and many other conditions are most likely to die during early morning hours (4-7 am), when their breathing is the heaviest, body oxygenation is critically low, and the CP is the shortest (about 5 seconds or less). You can investigate relevant quotes and observations of western medical doctors on the webpage "Morning Hyperventilation" (http://www.normalbreathing.com/index-MorningHV.php) or by watching my YouTube video-clip "How we breathe in the morning".

Most people also experience the shortest CPs during early morning hours and feel worst in the morning after waking up. Practical observations of Buteyko breathing teachers have confirmed that, indeed, in most people, up to 80% or more, their CPs significantly drops (up to 3-7 seconds or even more) during the night.

There are many causes that contribute to this Morning Hyperventilation effect. However, the very first aim for each person is to identify the presence and extent of this problem. How? Measure your CP immediately after waking up in the morning. As soon as you open your eyes, before getting out of the bed, do the stress- free breath holding time test. Have a ticking or other clock or watch nearby to help you define your breathing rate during last hours of sleep. The MCP (morning control pause) is the most important parameter of your physiological health.

4.3 Buteyko Table of Health Zones

Based on hundreds of medical studies, it is possible to suggest that the following effects take place with the progression of a chronic disease:
- we breathe more air (minute ventilation increases)
- breathing frequency becomes higher
- breathing becomes deeper (tidal volume increases)
- CO_2 content in blood decreases
- CP becomes shorter
- body oxygenation decreases
- heart rate increases, etc.

These effects are reflected in the **Buteyko Table of Health Zones**.

Amazing DIY Breathing Device

Health state	Type of breathing	Degree	Pulse, beats/min	Breathing frequency/min	CO2 in alveoli, %	AP, s	CP, s	MP, s
Super-health	Shallow	5	48	3	7.5	16	180	210
		4	50	4	7.4	12	150	190
		3	52	5	7.3	9	120	170
		2	55	6	7.1	7	100	150
		1	57	7	6.8	5	80	120
Normal	Normal	-	60	8	6.5	4	60	90
Disease	Deep	-1	65	10	6.0	3	50	75
		-2	70	12	5.5	2	40	60
		-3	75	15	5.0	-	30	50
		-4	80	20	4.5	-	20	40
		-5	90	26	4.0	-	10	20
		-6	100	30	3.5	-	5	10

Table comments: Pulse – heart rate in 1 minute (all parameters are measured at rest); Rf – respiratory frequency in one minute (number of inhalations or exhalations in one minute); % CO2 - %CO2 in alveoli of the lungs (*or arterial blood if there is no mismatch); AP - the Automatic Pause or natural delay in breathing after exhalation (*during unconscious breathing); CP - the Control Pause, breath holding time after usual exhalation and until first distress; WP - Willful Pause, breath holding time from the first distress until the limit (after it, make frequent, but small inhalations while breathing through a slightly pinched nose); MP (the Maximum Pause, the sum of the CP and WP.

* Note about pulse: Not all people have greatly increased heart rates, as is provided by this table, when parameters are at the bottom of the table or their CPs are low. Some categories of people with less than 20 second CP can have a resting pulse of around 60 - 70. However, increased heart rate for lower CPs is a feature of, for example, heart patients and patients with severe asthma. During the 1960's, when conducting his research, and later, Buteyko and his colleagues applied the Buteyko breathing retraining program mainly for heart and asthma patients, who were mostly hospitalized with frequent deficiencies in blood cortisol levels.

/ This version is based on Buteyko KP, The method of volitional elimination of deep breathing [English translation of the Small Buteyko Manual], Voskresensk, 1994.

Dr. Buteyko developed this table during 1960s, after analyzing hundreds of sick and healthy people in his respiratory laboratory, and presented it during his Lecture for the leading scientists at the Moscow State University in 1969. The Table reflects the health of his numerous hospitalized and severely sick patients, who started their journey for health at the very bottom of the table and climbed up, sometimes to the very top of the table.

The middle row of the table corresponds to normal health. Below this row are 7 zones corresponding to disease. The borders for these zones are given by 7 rows (from normal down to "minus 6-th" degree). Five zones of super-health are above the middle row. Let us start from the very bottom of this table and work up.

Terminally sick and critically ill patients during acute stages

The lowest row of this table corresponds to severely sick and terminally ill patients in critical conditions. When people are at the risk of dying, the table predicts over 100 beats per minute for their heart rate, over 30 breaths per minute for respiratory frequency, less than 3.5% CO_2 in the alveoli of the lungs. The CP (Control Pause or stress-free breath holding time after usual exhalation) is less than 5 seconds.

Terminally sick and critically ill patients in more stable conditions

The next row from the bottom corresponds to severely sick and terminally ill patients in stable conditions.

Typical heart rates of such people are above 90 beats per minute (sitting at

rest). Respiratory rate (or breathing frequency) is above 26 breaths per minute at rest. A CO_2 concentration in alveoli of the lungs is no more than 4%. There is no automatic pause (period of no breathing after exhalation). The Control Pause is less than 10 seconds, while the Maximum Pause is less than 20 seconds. (Numerous medical studies confirmed that over 90% of patients with chronic diseases indeed die in conditions of severe hyperventilation, while their heart rate and respiratory frequency become much higher than the norms.

Quotes and exact numbers from such studies can be found on my website in relation to heart disease, asthma, cancer, and many other conditions.)

These patients usually require numerous types of medication to prevent their multiple symptoms and complaints. Due to heavy labored breathing, dyspnea, and low body oxygenation at rest, walking is hard and climbing stairs is often impossible. Most of the time is spent in bed, since even sitting requires effort.

Sleep is dreadful since breathing and symptoms get much worse after transition into a horizontal position.

Early morning hours (4-7 am) is the time when these patients are most likely to die from heart attack, stoke, asthma attack, or complications from cancer, diabetes, and many other pathologies.

Patients with moderate degree of their disease

The next row ("minus 4-th" degree of health) corresponds to patients whose life is not threatened at the moment, but their main concern are symptoms. People with mild asthma, heart disease, diabetes, initial stages of cancer, and many other chronic disorders are all in this zone. Taking medication is the normal feature for most of these people.

As we see from the table, heart rate for these patients varies from 80 to 90 beats per minute. Breathing frequency is between 20 and 26 breaths per minute (the medical norm is 12, while doctor Buteyko's norm is 8 breaths per minute at rest). CO_2 concentration in alveoli of the lungs is between 4.0 and 4.5%. The CP is between 10 and 20 seconds.

Physical exercise is very hard, since even fast walking results in very heavy breathing through the mouth, exhaustion, and worsening of symptoms. Complains about fatigue are normal. All these symptoms are often so debilitating that they interfere with normal life and the ability to work, analyze information, care about others, etc. Living in the chronic state of stress and being preoccupied with one's own miserable health are normal, while efficiency and performance in various areas (science, arts, sports, etc.) are compromised. Sitting in armchairs or soft couches is the most favorite posture.

Parameters of these people get worse during early morning hours with corresponding worsening of symptoms. Many sufferers get less than 10 seconds for the morning CP with all effects accompanying the last stage of the disease.

Most modern people

Most modern healthy people have between 20 and 30 second CP. Hence, they are going to be in the third row from the bottom ("minus 3-rd" degree of health). While there is no need for taking medication in this zone, numerous health pathologies are frequent. This relates to gastrointestinal disorders (gastritis, IBS, IBD, etc.), musculoskeletal problems (arthritis, osteoporosis, etc.), hormonal and metabolic problems (mild obesity, light diabetes), initial stages of cancer, and many others.

Standing for many hours is hard and they prefer to sit for most part of the day. Physical performance after meals is very poor since respiratory and cardiovascular parameters can shift to the lower zone. The level of energy and physical desire to work are low. The over-excited brain easily invents excuses for laziness. Morning parameters are much worse (less than a 20 second CP) with all effects that are present for this zone.

Normal health

As we continue to climb up the table, the next row corresponds to the norms. The row "minus 2" reflects international norms for breathing: breathing frequency of 12 breaths per minute; 5.5 % for CO_2

concentrations in the alveoli of the lungs (about 41 mm Hg); 40 second CP and 70 beats per minute for heart rate. People with normal health naturally have a so called "automatic pause" or period of no breathing (total relaxation of all respiratory muscles after each exhalation) during their unconscious breathing. The duration of the automatic pause is about 2 seconds.

People with normal health are able to run with strictly nasal breathing, safely take a cold shower (if they follow certain other rules), have good quality sleep, and are reasonably able to function on the social level (family, community, workplace, etc.).

Buteyko norms

Dr. Buteyko suggested his own standards for health so that one can be free from about 200 chronic conditions. As we see in the table, healthy people should have a breathing frequency of no more than 8 breaths per minute at rest, more than 60 second CP, over 6.5% CO_2, less than 60 beats per min for heart rate, and at least 4 seconds for the automatic pause.

At this stage people enjoy and even crave physical activity. They are full of energy (when they have a normal blood glucose level). Standing throughout the day is easy and natural. Sleep is less than 5 hours and early morning parameters are not worse than evening ones. All tissues of the body are histologically normal (or in accordance with medical books), while chronic disorders are impossible.

Stages that correspond to super-health

Buteyko also identified 5 stages that correspond to super-health. Transition to the next row above the norm triggers certain biochemical processes and the appearance of lost abilities of the human body, including ability to digest wider varieties of fibers, painless childbirth, production of antibodies in saliva that prevent cavities and the formation of plague (no need to visit dentists 1-2 times every year), and some other effects.

Buteyko generalized this table to a wide variety of conditions (heart disease, cancer, diabetes, asthma, and many others). He considered this table as an important discovery since he applied for a patent. His patent application is provided below.

RUSSIA (19)RU (11)99114075 (13)A (51) IPC7 **A61B5/00**

FEDERAL SERVICE FOR INTELLECTUAL PROPERTY,

Patents and Trademarks

(21), (22) Application:**99114075/14, 23.06.1999**

(43) Date of publication of application:**27.04.2001**

Address for correspondence: **121609, Moscow, Osennyi Boulevard, 11, (609 office), Company "CEP"**

(71) Applicant (s): **Veltistova Elena, Buteyko Konstantin Pavlovich (UA)**

(72) Author (s): **Veltistova Elena, Buteyko Konstantin Pavlovich (UA)**

(54)**METHOD OF ASSESSMENT OF HUMAN HEALTH**

(57) Abstract:

1. The method of assessing human health, including the definition of the parameters of functional systems and calculation of health indicators based on the above parameters other than those that form the contingent of the surveyed people who determine the parameter information by measuring the breath holding time of the person after a usual exhalation before the first inhalation without following disturbances in breathing, and then determine and record the basic parameters of main functional systems, and each of them is compared with the informational parameter of the investigated person and obtain the parameter, which is a marker of major

functional systems and / or indicator of human health, create a method to assess health through establishment of the scale, while comparing the actual values of each parameter of health survey with the normal value, and based on the received data, health groups can be formed.

2. The method, according to Paragraph 1, but is different in that the scale of health has five categories with a positive sign that characterize the health status of people with different levels of super-endurance and seven categories with a negative sign, which characterize the state of poor health and / or disease in humans with varying degrees of disease severity.

5. How to increase CO2 and CP

5.1 Methods suggested by K. P. Buteyko

There were 2 methods or types of exercise suggested by Dr. Buteyko in order to temporarily boost CO2 content in the human body: 1) physical exercise; and 2) reduced breathing exercise.

During these activities CO2 content in the lungs, blood and other cells is higher than at rest and we get a stronger desire to breathe (air hunger). If we are able to tolerate this air hunger and relax for a certain time (from 5 minutes to about 2 hours), our body triggers the adaptation of the breathing centre to lighter breathing and higher CO2 concentrations in cells and tissues after the session. It is not the activity itself, but rather the after-effects of the activity that have to be analyzed for health benefits. When breathing becomes lighter, the final CP (Control Pause after the breathing session or physical exercise) is higher, indicating favorable adaptations of the respiratory centre. (Note that the CP usually does not increase after rigorous physical exercise. Physical exercise has a definite positive effect only on the next morning CP, which is the main parameter of health for the Buteyko method.)

5.2 Breathing devices

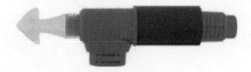

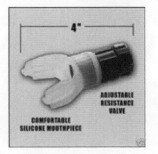

Any breathing device or an apparatus that resists to air flow and/or traps part of the inhaled air for the next inhalation will change the air composition in the alveoli of the lungs and blood. If the person does not try deliberate overbreathing and can relax instead of panic, then any device or apparatus will increase inhaled CO_2 (hypercapnia) and reduce inhaled O_2 content (hypoxia) producing positive effects on all systems of the human organism.

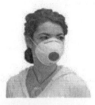

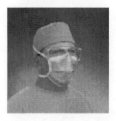

Consider a simple dust mask and a surgical mask. Both breathing devices create resistance to air flow and trap some exhaled air with very large CO_2 content. Breathing becomes slower and slightly deeper, but the body CO_2 content gets higher. (Nasal breathing increase the body CO_2 content in comparison with mouth breathing due to the same principle: greater resistance to air flow.) Hence, alveolar CO_2 gets slightly higher, while O_2 concentration is reduced.

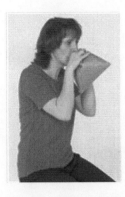

Similar effects (higher CO2 and hypoxia in the lungs with subsequent adaptation of the breathing centre) takes place during paper rebreathing, a popular technique known for 2-3 centuries and used by young artists in theaters before performance in order to prevent nervousness and stage fear and to reduce panic.

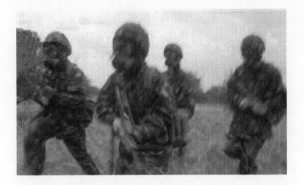

Another type of exercise, with large temporary CO2 increase, is running with gas masks (those heavy gas masks with carbon filters which are used in the military services). During Soviet times there were many legendary stories from young rookies about their dramatic health improvements after having daily runs (up to 10 km!), while wearing such breathing devices. Obviously, if one would be able to tolerate such an ordeal, it should lead to large changes in the direction of less breathing and better health.

From a physiological viewpoint, when using these breathing devices we tolerate higher arterial CO2 levels than arterial CO2 values present at rest. The longer the use of the device and the larger the change, the higher the final change in the arterial CO_2 after the session. Which devices are going to produce stronger effects? Clearly, the effects of a dust mask, surgical mask and paper bag are quite small since we hardly notice any air hunger. However, when we exercise and use, for example, a "PowerLung" or gas mask, while running,

we experience stronger air hunger. Both devices create strong resistance to our breathing. Hence, the effects of these devices during physical exercise can be more lasting.

5.3 Are deep breathing and mouth breathing always bad?

"And finally one should not confuse the following concepts: we are speaking about breathing, which goes on day and night, about our basal breathing, foundation of life. Meanwhile, the system of yogi has separate breathing exercises. Therefore, it is practically unimportant for us how and what you do: feet upwards or downwards, through the right or left nostril, or by right or left side. We are interested in where you will arrive as a result of these exercises. If carbon dioxide increases, and breathing decreases, with each day, then this will ensure the transition of man into a super-endurance state..." Dr. Buteyko's lecture in the Moscow State University on 9 December 1969

"... *The diver does about 100 dives 2 minutes each; for 200 minutes or 3 hours he is under water [every day]. This is most active work. But this is not that important. It is how he breathes the other 21 hours, instead of those 3 hours. If he breathes deeply, then he will be severely sick and will die. And if he breathes normally, he will somehow endure 3 hours. The key is not in the dive, but in the way the person breathes day and night. First, what is the basal breathing?*" Dr. Buteyko's lecture in the Moscow State University on 9 December 1969

Is deep breathing (or large minute ventilation) always dangerous or disadvantageous for health? During physical exercise our breathing rate is also very large (up to 100-150 L/min), but CO_2 in the lungs and arterial blood increases, as in the case of nasal breathing during physical exercise, causing gradual adaptation of the breathing centre to higher CO_2 values. (This is the main mechanism, according to Dr. Buteyko why physical exercise is good for our health.) Buteyko also taught us that we are biochemical machines, not mechanical ones. In his words, a rigid approach to breathing ("any deep breathing is bad") is silly. Most importantly, we should see what is going on with the CO_2 content in the human organism after training. Hence, we should find changes in the CP before and after the breathing session.

The same ideas should be applied to mouth breathing. During mouth breathing in normal life, alveolar CO_2 content drops and nitric oxide is not inhaled in the lungs. Sick people, due to abnormal parameters of their breathing pattern (fast exhalations and absence of the autonomic pause), have greatly reduced NO (nitric oxide) intake. With healthy people, main NO accumulation takes place during automatic pauses so that they can inhale it in after the automatic pause.

Let us consider what is going on with these parameters (CO_2 and NO) during mouth breathing through some device. If the device can trap a portion of the air exhaled, then this CO_2 can be inhaled in during the next inspiration. Hence, breathing devices (paper bags, gas masks, dust masks, etc.) increase CO_2 content in the blood and in all cells of the human body.

If the person does active inhalations through the mouth, while wearing or using the breathing device, then a small portion of the air (about 5-10% at least) will be inhaled through the nose involuntarily. Hence, the person will inhale NO that has been accumulated in the nasal passages during the automatic pause and slow inhalation through the mouth. If the person uses nasal clips, nitric oxide will be retained in sinuses and most likely get diffused through mucosal surfaces into the bloodstream. (Heart patients normally take nitroglycerine, which is converted in the body into NO, sublingually, i.e. under the tongue. It should not be a problem for NO to diffuse through mucosal membranes.)

Therefore, mouth breathing through the device should not produce any negative effects even during the breathing session. Finally, when various breathing exercises are practiced, it is necessary to consider the after-effects of these breathing exercises on the main parameters of the human organism: most of all, changes

in the CP and heart rate. This is exactly what Buteyko taught us: consider changes in basal breathing or breathing that is going on unconsciously, the remaining 23 hours per day.

5.4 Factors for success: knowledge, direction and attitude

Clear understanding of the goals of breathing retraining is also necessary for success. A student may practice the best breathing exercises for 1-2 hours every day, but if this student, after a breathing session, goes to neighbors and spends 2 hours talking non-stop about feeling great after the session, and thus hyperventilating, he or she will not get any positive changes in their breathing, since the goal of the breathing retraining is to change the breathing pattern or our unconscious (basal) breathing.

For those students, who learned the foundations of the Buteyko method and are aware about CO2 effects, body oxygenation, CP measurement, and main life-style factors, the result will be totally different since they will try, even unconsciously, to maintain light easy breathing patterns after the session. It is not the name of the device, or type of the session, or miracles hidden in the device, but what the student is going to do with his or her breathing after the session that also defines the lasting changes or final outcomes.

The general emotions or attitudes of the person towards breathing retraining, including perception of one's own abilities, skills, body, and many other related factors, will greatly influence the general progress. Simplicity, a business-oriented approach, modesty, and perseverance will definitely help to have better long- term results.

5.5 Restrictions, limits, and temporary contraindications

For people with transplanted organs

You should not have more than 30 seconds for your CP (preferably less than 27 s) at any time of the day to prevent rejection of the transplanted organs. When the CP gets more than 30 seconds (it corresponds to transition to the next health zone according to the Buteyko Table of Health Zones), the immune system becomes more sensitive to foreign tissues and cells and can launch an attack on these tissues in the attempt to repair them.

For people in life-threatening situations

Modern EM (Emergency Medicine) professionals developed many successful and useful methods and techniques for people in critical care and life-threatening states. Breathing retraining cannot replace these techniques (CPR, breathing pure oxygen, etc.) when people are unconscious or are unable to have a good control of their actions. Breathing exercises cannot quickly stop progression of metastasizing cancer. **Acute stages (exacerbations) of life-threatening conditions** (infarct, stroke, cardiac ischemia, severe asthma attack, metastasizing cancer, septic shock, multiple organ failure, near-death experience, etc.)

Later, when one's state is stabilized, the person can start breathing exercises and apply those exercises that correspond to their new health state.

For people with acute bleeding injuries and brain traumas
Hyperventilation is a normal and useful reaction to bleeding injuries. Reduced CO_2 content in the blood decreases blood flow to vital organs and other tissues of the human body. This prevents excessive blood losses and can save one's life. Emergency professionals even coined a term "permissive hyperventilation" that is used for people with, for example, brain trauma. Hence, one should not reduce or

restrict their breathing in cases of existing brain traumas and acute bleeding injuries.

For people with blood clots

Reduced breathing dilates arteries and arterioles and makes blood thinner so that an existing blood clot could get loose and travel via the blood. The released clot may block blood flow through the artery leading to the brain or heart muscle and cause death. Hence, a person with a blood clot will benefit only from defensive measures in relation to breathing retraining (prevention of CP drops due to mouth breathing, sleeping on one's back, correct posture, etc.). These defensive activities prevent periods of hyperventilation that make blood thicker and the clot larger. Later, when the clot is dissolved or removed, the person can follow the program of breathing retraining adjusted to their new health state.

For people with loss of CO2 sensitivity

Loss of CO2 sensitivity takes place due to near death experience, carotid bodies removed, denervation of respiratory muscles (there are medical publications with abnormally high breath holding test results for all these situations), and life-style and environmental causes for genetically predisposed people (lack of deep stages of sleep, cortisol deficiency, calcium deficiency, EFA deficiency, magnesium deficiency, zinc deficiency, too low blood glucose, hyper and hypothermia, allergic reactions, etc.).

Practically, the last case (life-style and environmental causes) is the most frequent one. It can be episodic or chronic (for days or weeks). Many heart patients (they are predisposed to loss of CO2 sensitivity) can be driven into this state, if they use pauses, even the CP only, indiscriminately. The CP reflects their health, but they can feel worse after it; and repetitive pauses or just one MP can lead them in a state with no CO2 sensitivity.

When the person has experienced loss of CO2 sensitivity, their CPs do not reflect their health anymore. Generally, the CP reflects personal health for other 97% of people, but these people (with sensitivity to CO2 absent) can have disproportionally high CPs. For example, a student has 45 second CP (can be even up to 50-60 s), but his other symptoms are: irregular and visible upper chest breathing, high blood pressure (or asthma), poor and long sleep (over 8 hours), low energy level, etc, so that his clinical picture corresponds to about 15-20 second CP.

Such students require restoration of normal environmental and other parameters in order to restore normal CO2 sensitivity. Depending on the severity of the current state, these students require a special program based on their ability to have positive changes after a particular exercise.

For example, in the most severe cases a simple relaxation/meditation exercise (with no breathing control) can cause higher heart rates and lower CPs. When the condition is less severe, students can successfully meditate or practice relaxation only, but any attempt to reduce breathing or to breathe through a breathing device could lead to a worsened health state.

For pregnant women

The main danger for pregnancy is spontaneous abortion during a cleansing reaction due to very fast CP progress. For example, a pregnant woman starts with about 12-15 second CP and achieves 35-40 second CP in 4-6 days due to intensive breathing retraining. The immune system becomes highly sensitive to abnormal tissues and is able to reject transplanted organs, as we considered above. Similarly, the immune system at higher CPs can easily reject an embryo at the state when it is not yet attached to the womb of the mother (the first trimester of the pregnancy). The chances of spontaneous abortion are much higher, if the growing embryo accumulated medical drugs or if the mother had been taking medication before and after getting pregnant.

In order to prevent this, women should have a defensive program of breathing retraining based on prevention of CP losses (episodes of hyperventilation) due to overeating, mouth breathing, poor posture, morning hyperventilation, etc. The rate of CP progress should be limited:

- for women who used medical drugs or were exposed to toxic chemicals by 2 seconds in one week

- for other pregnant women by 3 seconds in one week.

For type 2 diabetics

Intensive breathing sessions and quick CP growth increase the organism's sensitivity to circulating insulin and increase production of its own insulin due to better perfusion and oxygenation of the pancreas. This can happen due to a single breathing session or due to a fast CP growth within hours or days of first lessons. Hence, taking the same insulin dose can easily lead to hypoglycemic shock, which is potentially fatal. In order to prevent these complications, the student should:

1) eat a small snack immediately after a breathing session to prevent a drop in blood glucose level

2) adjust daily insulin requirements to their current state by having good blood glucose control (periodic measurements), consulting their GP or family physician or endocrinologist about decreased blood glucose values, and asking them about reduced insulin intake.

Most diabetics, when they have the cooperation of their doctors, can safely decrease their insulin intake about 2 times after they start their program of breathing retraining described below.

For heart disease, migraine headaches, or panic attacks patients
Depending on the severity and type of the condition and some other factors, many of these patients can worsen their health state if they try very intensive breathing sessions accompanied by quick CO_2 increase. For example, breath holds can trigger negative cardiovascular changes. Note that other groups of people can do

breath holds without any negative effects, but blood vessels of heart patients can constrict due to sudden hypoxia. This effect was known to Dr. K. Buteyko who described it in his medical publication in the 1960's.

Therefore, when these patients have less than 20 second CP, they have 2 choices.

1. Inhale air through the nose and exhale through the breathing device

2. Breathe in and out through the device but use a device with a very small volume for the plastic tube (no more than 50 ml). This can be achieved by using a very narrow plastic bottle. In both cases, their breathing should remain regular (no breath holds).

Later, when their CPs are more than 20 seconds, these students can try a common breathing session with no air hunger and a comfortable state of well-being during the exercise. When they get over 30 second CP, no restrictions are necessary and they can join the main group in further breathing normalization.

Heart disease (aortic aneurysms; angina pectoris; arrhythmia; atherosclerosis (plaque buildup); cardiomyopathy; ciliary arhythmia (cardiac fibrillation); chest pain (angina pectoris); high cholesterol; chronic ischemia; congenital heart disease; congestive heart failure; coronary artery disease; endocarditis; extrasystole; heart murmurs; hypertension; hypertrophic cardiomyopathy; pericarditis; postmyocardial infarction; stroke; tachnycardia)

Migraine headaches and panic attacks

For people with respiratory disorders involving lungs

These groups of people should be gentle in relation to their damaged lungs tissue. Intensive mechanical stimulation of their lungs (in terms of amplitude and velocity of inhalation and exhalations) during initial stages of learning should be avoided. Later, they can gradually increase these parameters. This relates to people with:

Respiratory disorders involving the lungs (asthma, bronchitis, COPD, emphysema, cystic fibrosis, pneumonia, tuberculosis; pulmonary edema; etc.)

Hence, they should avoid any fast inhalation and exhalations, as well as maximum inflations and deflations of their lungs. All exercises are done in a comfortable way with good care for the current abilities of their lungs.

6. How to make and try DIY breathing device

6.1 Required parts and assembling

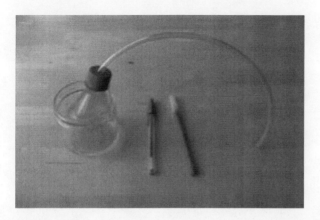

The image on the right side shows a DIY breathing device that is ready to use. (The pens are there to show the scale of the objects and for recording your progress every day.) The required parts to construct your personal DIY breathing device are:

1) A glass jar or plastic container;

2) Upper part of a plastic bottle;

3) A cap with a small round hole from the same plastic bottle;

4) Vinyl tubing (20-25 cm long or even more; 4-10 mm in inner diameter depending on your CP).

Let us consider all these parts and their parameters in more detail.

A glass jar or plastic container

The glass jar will have a small amount of water (about 20-40 ml) at the bottom so that you can inhale and exhale while breathing only through water. (This device can be used as an inhaler.)

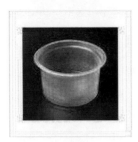

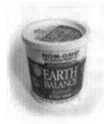

Instead of 500 ml glass jar, you can use a plastic container. Two examples are shown on the left. Make sure that their bottom is quite flat and that their bottom surface area is not very large. If the surface area is too large, then, during inhalation most of the water will be collected in the plastic bottle, and water drops could easily move into the vinyl tube and reach your mouth. There is no danger, but it is better to focus on the breathing and not worry about the water getting

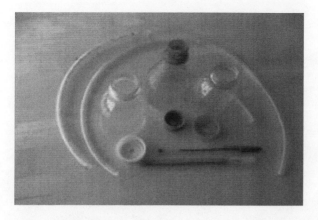

Let us now focus on the other parts of the device. These parts are shown here on the right.

Upper part of a plastic bottle

In most households, it is easy to find an ordinary plastic bottle (about 500-600 ml are the most popular ones). This bottle has to be cut along a circular diameter so that the top part of the bottle will have about 200-250 ml of volume left.

Do not try to make the cut perfect. Sometimes, the perfect cut will result in the "sealing effect". You will not be able to take an inhale if the bottom of your breathing device perfectly matches the contact surface of the container.

Warning. Since ordinary kitchen knives and scissors are often blunt and can slip under pressure, it can be dangerous to use them without some preparation as you could easily hurt yourself. However, if you make a tiny initial hole (or several holes) using a needle or a safety pin, then it will be much safer and easier to cut the bottle using scissors.

Cap with a hole from the same plastic bottle

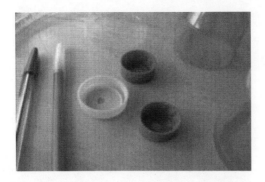

This image on the left shows 3 caps with round holes in them. To make a simpler device, you have to drill a hole that has a diameter slightly less than the outer diameter of the tube. If you manage to make such a match, the tube will solidly stay / sit in the bottle cap. Generally, this job will require a drill.

Warning. Some plastic bottle caps are very hard and thick. You could easily hurt your arms or fingers, if you use knives or scissors. However, if you manage to make a tiny hole using a nail and a hammer or a corkscrew, then it will be easier to expand the hole.

If you cannot make the hole of the optimum size in the cap and your hole is too large, you may use tape to connect the tube and the cap of the bottle, so that it looks like this (see the image below).

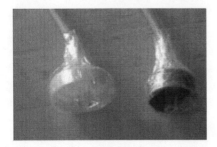

Vinyl tube

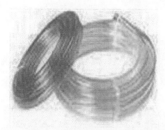

A piece of clear vinyl tube (used for drinking water) can be bought in home hardware stores. Do not buy dark tubes that are used for gardening or other purposes. It should be light, clean and clear vinyl tubing as shown on the left. The required length of the tube is 20-25 cm. It is better to buy 3 or 4 different types of vinyl tubing and make 3-4 breathing devices so that you can try them all and choose the most suitable one depending on your health state. It usually costs less than 1 US$/CAN$ for 1 foot of tube in North America and less than 2 Euro in Europe.

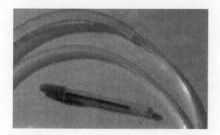

When you have different devices and tubes with different diameters, you can easily try and even modify your DIY devices since the tubes can be inserted inside each other with no trouble. Hence, any device with a wider tube can be made more difficult to use if you insert a short piece or narrower tube into a free end of a tube that is a part of the existing device. The picture on the right shows how 2 pieces of tubing can be easily connected with each other to form a combined tube (the upper one).

If you have only about 10-15 second CP or less, you will require a tube with a large diameter (about 8-10 mm is the optimum dimension to start with). For people with higher initial CP (20 seconds or more), try to find a narrower tube (6-8 mm in inner diameter). You will have a better understanding of your optimum breathing device after you've practiced your first breathing sessions and got comfortable with your own creations: your first DIY breathing devices.

When you start trying your DIY devices, choose the one which is not the easiest, but the one that you find yourself the most comfortable to breathe through. If you spend about 3-4 days using this easy and comfortable approach, you will learn how your body reacts to your attempts to retrain your breathing.

6.2 Physiological effects

Changes in inhaled air composition due to the DIY breathing device

When we breathe only through the device (inhalations and exhalations), there are changes in the air composition that enters our lungs. Indeed, during our exhalation, part of the exhaled air is trapped in the plastic bottle. This air in the bottle has much higher CO_2 concentration (up to about 5-6% in most practical situations) and much less oxygen (about 14-16%). Normal air has about 20% oxygen and 0.03% CO_2. Hence, during our next inhalation this trapped air mixes with fresh air and this air composition (more CO_2 and less O_2) enters into our lungs. The approximate composition of the inhaled air is provided in this Table.

Inhaled air during breathing sessions		
Gas composition parameter	Inhaled normal air	Inhaled air during breathing sessions
CO2 content	0.03% CO2	1-2% CO2
O2 content	20% O2	18-19% O2

The exact composition of the inhaled air is difficult to predict because it depends on many parameters:
1) volume of trapped air in the plastic bottle (the larger this volume,

the higher the inhaled CO_2 and the lower the exhaled O_2);
2) amplitude of breathing (it is called tidal volume);
3) breathing frequency (it is considered in the next section);
4) metabolic rate (or CO_2-generation rate).

Those people, who inhale through the nose and exhale through the device, do not use air that is trapped in the device for their breathing. However, since they try to make longer exhalations, their lungs naturally accumulate more CO_2 and have less O_2. Hence, they experience a similar physiological effect, but to a smaller degree. Therefore, using the DIY device is a type of **intermittent hypercapnic hypoxic training**. Similar effects (more CO_2 and less O_2 in inhaled air) take place during Buteyko breathing exercises and pranayama (a slow deep breathing exercise from hatha yoga). Hypoxic training (less O_2) without hypercapnia takes place when athletes and other people have their training sessions and/or live at high altitude (1,500-3,000 m high).

DBC (duration of the breathing cycle) and breathing frequency

During normal breathing (official medical international norm) we breathe 12 breaths per minute at rest. Hence, the duration of the breathing cycle is 5 seconds. 5 seconds times 12 makes 60 seconds or one minute. When using the breathing device, DBC (duration of the breathing cycle) varies among people. The CP is the main factor that defines one's DBC.

For example, if somebody has about a 50-60 second CP, this person can breathe through the device very slowly or only about 1 breath per minute. Their DBC can be about 60 seconds. Why is it so? If we think about minute ventilation, or amount of air we breathe in one minute, a person with 60 second CP breathes only about 4 L/min at rest. This is less than the modern medical norm, which is 6 L/min (liters per minute). When breathing through the device with maximum diaphragmatic inhalation and exhalation, such a person can use about 3 L of fresh air per one breath. Hence, this person is going to breathe little less (3 L/min instead of his usual 4 L/min) during a typical breathing session.

Let us now consider the breathing parameters of sick people. A typical body oxygenation of a sick person is 15 seconds and their typical minute ventilation is about 15 L per minute (see previous tables and graphs). When using this device, this sick person can also breathe a little less than before, for example, about 12 L/min. If this sick person takes 3 L of air per one inhalation (while using the DIYdevice), he will require 4 breaths per minute to have 12 L/min for his minute ventilation. Therefore, this person will require 4 breaths per one minute to get 12 L of air in the lungs in one minute. His DBC will be 15 seconds or, indeed, the same as his CP.

Hence, personal CP is the main factor that predicts the DBC. Some people, however, have larger lung capacity (up to 4 L or of air). Other people can have only about 2 l. Hence, lungs capacity will influence their DBC as well.

6.3 First easy and relaxed attempts

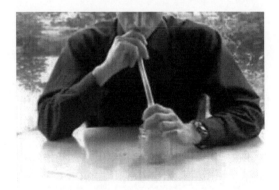

When your device is ready to use and your stomach is empty (no solid food in the stomach; water is ok), try to take several breaths so that you can experience its effects. (It is not the breathing session yet, which will be explained below.) As you can see on the left, one hand is gently pressing on the top of the plastic bottle and the other hand keeps the end of the tube in your mouth.

Take an active comfortable inhalation using your diaphragm (stomach or belly) only, and then exhale slowly and completely relaxing all your body muscles. Then again repeat the steps:

maximum comfortable inhalation followed by a relaxed complete exhalation. Make sure that you breathe primarily through the device: water bubbles are seen inside the bottle part during inhalations and outside it during exhalations. (As one may realize, water is used here as a feedback medium mainly. It helps us to see that we are actually breathing in and out through the device. Apart from that, it is known that very young children are fascinated by playing with water due to its almost alive behavior. This may even help you to relax better.)

6.4 Possible problems with your breathing device and their solutions

Water is spilling out of the container during exhalations. Your container is not tall enough or you may have too much water in the glass jar or the plastic container. Solution: find a taller container and use less water.

You cannot breathe for more than 2-3 minutes. Sometimes, a person can take only 3-5 breaths through the device and finds it too difficult to use. Try breathing more: deeper and/or more rapidly. If this is still the problem (an overwhelming sensation of air hunger), then the device may have too much resistance. Your tube is maybe too narrow or too long, or the volume of air in the bottle is too large. Solutions: you require a wider tube, or shorter tube, or less air volume in the bottle (trim the bottle at the bottom).

You cannot inhale since your plastic bottle perfectly fits the bottom of the container. This happens very rarely when your cut at the bottom of the plastic bottle is too smooth. Solutions: make some irregularities or tiny grooves on your bottle so that air can get in during your inhalations.

Too much water is getting into your mouth. This happens when the end of the vinyl tube is too close to water surface during inhalations. It can happen when the device is too low or there is too much water. If your container has a very large surface area, then there is too much water and most of the water is collected in the plastic bottle during inhalations. Solutions: reduce the amount of water you use or make a taller breathing device (use a narrower bottle).

You have difficulty breathing only with your mouth (involuntary breathing through the nose and inability to block nasal breathing). Some people, not many, regardless of their health and the CP, cannot breathe only through the mouth (even if they try) unless they pinch the nose. They will notice immediately that water bubbles appear only sporadically when they breathe through the device. In normal conditions, one should observe water bubbles either outside the bottle (during exhalations) or inside the bottle (during inhalations). Solutions: buy a nasal clip for swimming or pinch your nose with the thumb and index finger while holding the end of the vinyl tube in your mouth and keeping the tube between the remaining fingers of the same hand.

7 Requirements for breathing sessions

7.1 Empty stomach

The exercises are done strictly on an empty stomach (water is OK). Larger CO_2 concentrations provide more blood and oxygen for the GI system intensifying peristalsis. Many people today have inflammation in the stomach that they are unaware of, as recent western studies revealed. This inflammation can get worse due to intensification of peristalsis in the stomach and duodenum, if food is present there. (Imagine what could happen if somebody starts to vigorously rub skin areas which are already inflamed.) Having water in the stomach does not cause this problem.

7.2 Hydration

Acidification of blood due to increased CO_2 content triggers biological pH buffers in the blood. A part of this process is redistribution of ions in various compartments of the body (intracellular fluid, extra-cellular fluid, blood plasma, intestinal content, etc.). These processes may require additional water. Hence, drink if you get thirsty at any stage, even in the middle of the breathing session.

7.3 Thermoregulation

Find a comfortable place without draught, but not too warm. If your current CP is less than 20 seconds, keep yourself comfortably warm all the time. Overcooling is dangerous at this state. If your CP is above 20 seconds, try to have relatively cool conditions for breathing exercises. You may feel warm or even hot during the exercises. Some people start to sweat (perspire) when using the device. Therefore, be ready for that to happen and take steps to restore your thermal comfort: take some clothes off to normalize your heat exchange. If the place is too warm, it is often impossible to reduce breathing.

7.4 Clean and fresh air

While water in the container and especially moisture in the vinyl tube accumulate most air-born particles that are present in the inhaled air, it is still better to have good air quality in the place where you practice the breathing sessions. The place for exercises should have clean fresh air so that the student's nose is cold and moist, as it naturally happens outdoors.

7.5 Posture

Severely sick students with low initial CPs (less than 10 s) can do breathing exercises while lying, half-lying or sitting in a comfortable armchair with their backs supported. It is more important for them to have proper relaxation, since even light physical exertion due to sitting can significantly intensify their breathing.

When the CP is above 10 seconds, students should practice with their elbows and arms on the table, while sitting on the edge of a solid chair without using back support. The spine should be straight and erect. That is another crucial parameter for breathing normalization. It is important for the position of the diaphragm that the thighs are either horizontal or inclined downwards when in the sitting position. If the thighs are inclined upwards, as when sitting on a low chair, the diaphragm is compressed by the internal organs and it loses its mobility. Diaphragmatic breathing requires straight posture so that the diaphragm, instead of being compressed, is freely suspended and can easily be moved down and up.

Exceptions. Some people may suffer from back pain, when sitting up straight. If this is a case with you, you can lean on the back of a chair or find another solution so as to prevent back pain.

There is a test to check one's own posture. You only need a flat vertical surface (e.g., a wall or door).

The "wall test" for correct posture

Stand straight against a wall (or door) so that you can touch the wall with following 6 points on your body at the same time:
- both back sides of your shoes (2 points);
- your lowest vertebra (1 point);
- both your shoulder blades (2 points);
- the back of your head (1 point).

Some people find that they are looking too high when they try the "wall test". Probably they get used to looking down at the ground in front of them, but what is important is that this test helps to correct and restore the normal position of the spine so that breathing retraining is possible.

7.6 Diaphragmatic breathing

When one's CP is about 15-20 seconds, slouching means a 1-2 second CP decrease, while a straight spine can add 1-2 seconds to the CP. Those who continue to slouch are unable to get more than 30 second CP.

(Note that many modern people with a tendency to slouch, and especially when constipation is another symptom, require additional Mg (magnesium) supplementation. Mg is a powerful muscular relaxant and an additional factor to eliminate slouching.) When the CP gets up to about 40 seconds or more, correct posture becomes totally natural and does not require any conscious attention.

The simple mechanics of normal breathing at rest or how the diaphragm works The diaphragm, in a relaxed state (or after exhalation), has a shape of a cone or dome. During inhalation we stretch it in radial directions making it flatter: the upper part of the diaphragm moves down, while its sides move mostly in radial directions. For exhalations, we just relax the diaphragm and it returns (recoils) back to its original position. Chest muscles are relaxed all the time. Try to visualize this process. Do you have diaphragmatic breathing at rest?

It is crucial for health to have diaphragmatic breathing at rest, during sleep, and other activities with low metabolic rate. (The reasons and mechanisms are explained on the website www.NormalBreathing.com. The main reasons are normal blood oxygenation and natural drainage of the lymph nodes under the diaphragm is not possible with chest breathing.) Generally, when the CP is over 30 seconds, people naturally use their diaphragm for breathing at rest. When the CP is less than 20 seconds, since the diaphragm is a smooth muscle of the human body, it gets into a state of spasm due to CO_2 deficiency. As a result, most people switch to predominantly chest breathing. From 20 to 30 second CP is a transitory zone.

Most people have no problems with diaphragmatic breathing when breathing through the DIY device. However, some people, especially older and elderly ones, who have been chest-breathers for decades, may require additional exercises in order to develop their diaphragmatic breathing.

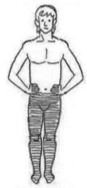

Exercise 1

Since we use almost the maximum amplitude of breathing, when using the DIY breathing device, it is relatively easy to have diaphragmatic breathing during breathing sessions. However, some people might be uncertain about their control of chest and diaphragmatic muscles. Then they should investigate these abilities and practice the simple breathing exercises described below.

Feeling the breath (3 simple exercises)

Exercise 1. Put the arms around your waist line (see the picture on the left), as if embracing yourself, and listen to your usual breathing for about 20-30 seconds. You will be able to detect the movements of the diaphragm, if you use it for breathing.

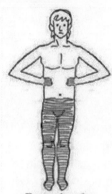

Exercise 2

Exercise 2. Put the arms slightly above the waist (about 10 cm or 4 inches higher) around your waist (see the picture on the right) so that you feel your lower ribs.

Listen to your usual breathing for about 20-30 seconds. You will be able to detect the movements of the rib cage and the diaphragm, if your arms are simultaneously on your lower ribs and on your belly. Take 2-3 slow deep breaths to have a more clear sensation about the dynamics of your breathing. Can you breathe using your belly only so that your rib cage does not move at all?

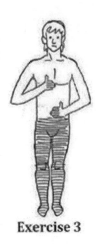

Exercise 3

Exercise 3. Put one of your arms on your belly (stomach) and another one higher, on your upper chest (see the picture on the left). Listen to your breathing again for about 20-30 seconds. Again take 2-3 slow deep breaths to feel your breathing in more detail. Can you breathe using your belly only so that your rib cage and upper arm do not move?

If you noticed that you do use your chest for breathing at rest, practice these exercises to develop abdominal breathing.

Developing diaphragmatic breathing (3 simple exercises)

Exercise 4. The same as the previous exercise: put one of your arms on your belly (stomach) and another one higher, on your upper chest (see the picture on the left above for Exercise 3). Try to move or push out your lower arm (which is on the belly button or navel) with your abdominal muscles. Create light resistance using this lower arm and keep your chest or rib cage relaxed. If it is still difficult to relax the chest, try the next exercise.

Exercise 5 (the exercise with books to acquire diaphragmatic breathing).

Take 2-3 medium weight books or one large phone book (e.g., yellow pages phone book) and lie down on your back with the books on your tummy. Focus on your breathing and change the way you breathe so that you can see that:

1) you can lift the books up about 2-3 cm (1 inch) with each inhalation and then relax to exhale (the books will go down);

2) your rib cage does not expand during inhalations.

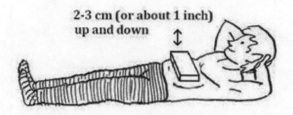

Repeat it for about 3-5 minutes before breathing sessions to reconnect your conscious brain with the diaphragm. You can practice this exercise for some days until you are sure that diaphragmatic breathing is the usual way to breathe during the breathing sessions. Once the CP is over 30 seconds, the spasmodic state of the diaphragm is naturally released (for some people with persistently tense diaphragm, magnesium can be an additional assisting factor) and it becomes the main muscle for breathing at rest.

If the diaphragm is still not the main muscle for your breathing and/or you have doubts about your ability to keep your chest relaxed during breathing exercises, apply this ultimate solution.

Exercise 6 A belt for diaphragmatic breathing)

You can use a strong belt to restrict your rib cage and "force" the diaphragm to be the main breathing muscle using the following technique.

Put a belt around your lower ribs (in the middle of the trunk) and buckle it tightly so that you cannot take a deep inhale using your rib cage or chest.

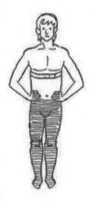

Now for slow deep inhalations your body needs to use your tummy (or abdomen). Try it. While leaving the belt for some minutes or even hours, you can acquire diaphragmatic breathing and corresponding sensations. This process is faster, if you focus your attention on your breathing. The focus of attention makes nervous links between your conscious mind and the diaphragm reinforced so that you can regain control of this muscle. Do not hyperventilate when you pay attention to your breathing! Breathe slowly and remain relaxed so that even if your inhales deepen, your CO_2 will not lessen.

7.7 A quiet place to focus one's attention

A session requires about 10-20 min of concentrated work without disturbances and interruptions. Being concentrated is important during initial stages of learning. Later, after many hours of practice, breathing exercises might be done while watching TV, reading, etc., but virtually all advanced students report better results when they are focused on their breathing and relaxation of body muscles.

7.8 A ticking clock or watches to monitor seconds

Amazing DIY Breathing Device

In order to measure your heart rate and CP and monitor your parameters of the breathing cycle (duration of inhalations and inhalations), you should have any device that shows seconds. It is even better, if, in addition, you have any device that generates a sound that is similar to a ticking clock. In this case you do not need to visually observe time, but you can hear clicks every second so that you easily count the durations of your inhalations and exhalations with minimum distraction.

8. First breathing sessions

8.1 Are you ready?

You are ready to go, if you:

● get the correct theoretical education about breathing, CO_2 effects, breath patterns, body oxygenation, the CP test, and influence of life style factors;

● make sure that all 7 preliminary requirements for breathing exercises, including no solid food in the stomach, are satisfied (see the previous chapter);

● do follow the additional suggestions for people who require a special approach to breathing retraining (restrictions, limits, and temporary contraindications section); then you can start your first practical lessons.

8.2 Remember your initial breathing

Focus on your breathing for 2-3 minutes at rest while sitting up straight. What do you feel? If the sensations are vague, take a deep slow in-breath and slowly exhale. Do you feel how the airflow goes through your

nostrils? Do you have any sensations at the back of your throat? Are there

any feelings about movement of air inside the chest and bronchi? What do you sense near your stomach? Try to remember these sensations so that you can compare them with your sensations after the breathing session. This will help you to understand and reinforce the direction in which your breathing is changing.

Measure your initial heart rate during a 30 second time interval and multiply this number by 2 so that you know your pulse (the number of heart beats in one minute). Measure your initial CP. Write down both numbers in your daily log. (The table for your daily log is explained and provided below.)

8.3 First 2-3 minutes or a "warm-up" period

You should adjust your program and

follow special suggestions (described above), if you have: Heart disease (aortic aneurysms; angina pectoris; arrhythmia; atherosclerosis (plaque buildup); cardiomyopathy; ciliary arhythmia (cardiac fibrillation); chest pain (angina pectoris); high cholesterol; chronic ischemia; congenital heart disease; congestive heart failure; coronary artery disease; endocarditis; extrasystole; heart murmurs; hypertension; hypertrophic cardiomyopathy; tachnycardia; pericarditis; postmyocardial infarction; stroke)

Migraine headaches and panic attacks

Respiratory disorders involving lungs (asthma, bronchitis, COPD, emphysema, cystic fibrosis, pneumonia, tuberculosis; pulmonary edema; etc.)

Presence of transplanted organs

Pregnancy

Brain traumas

Acute bleeding injuries

Blood clots

Acute stages (exacerbations) or life-threatening conditions (infarct, stroke, cardiac ischemia, septic shock, etc.)

Insulin-dependent diabetes (type 2 diabetes) Loss of CO_2 sensitivity

During the first 2-3 minutes your goal is to find a comfortable breathing pattern for this session. Make active and maximum inhalations using your diaphragm (or belly or stomach) through your breathing device while keeping your chest relaxed. The duration of inhalation mainly depends on the diameter and length of the tube. If your CP is less than 20 seconds, your duration of inhalation should be no more than one third of your CP. If your CP is higher (over 20 s), 6-7 seconds for duration of your maximum inhalation is a good choice. After this maximum and active inhalation, your goal is to relax and make a complete exhalation. How quickly or for how long? This depends primarily on your current CP, lung volume, power of your respiratory muscles, and your current metabolic rate. You may simply breathe in and out through the device and follow the sensations of your body so that you feel comfortable all the time. People with lower CPs should breathe quite fast. Otherwise, they feel as if they are suffocated. People with higher CPs can breathe slower.

You will discover after several breathing sessions that your BCD (breathing cycle duration), when using the breathing device, is close and directly proportional to your current CP. For example, if your CP is around 10 seconds, then you should exhale quickly (during about 6-9 seconds) since your BCD (breathing cycle duration) will be close to your current CP. If you have about 25-30 second CP now, your exhale can be much more relaxed and longer in time (up to about 20-25 s).

When you make 5-6 inhalations and exhalations, you should be able to find a comfortable pattern of breathing for this session. If you have a ticking clock nearby, then you can easily figure out that it takes you, for example, 3 seconds to inhale (using your diaphragm) and 7 seconds for exhalation. Then your BCD is easy to find: 3 seconds + 7 seconds = 10 seconds.

If you feel air hunger or are suffocating and cannot continue, use another device with a wider tube and reduced volume of the plastic bottle. If you feel that a wider tube is too easy for you, chose a narrower one, but remember about comfort for your first breathing sessions.

8.4 The main part of the lesson

After you have found your comfortable BCD (breathing cycle duration), the goal is to maintain this pattern of breathing for next 15-20 minutes (for adults). Assume that during "warm-up" you could go on with 3 seconds "in" and 7 seconds "out" for several breaths up to 3-4 minutes in total. Afterwards, you should continue the same pattern (3 seconds "in" and 7 seconds "out") for the rest of the breathing session.

Note 1. If during the session you find that it is easy to have longer exhalation, you may increase your inhalations provided that you indeed feel totally comfortable with it. For example, imagine that you started with 4 seconds for inhalation and 10 seconds for exhalation. Your initial BCD was therefore 14 seconds during first 2-3 minutes. It is suggested above that you should stick with the same breathing pattern and BCD (14 s) for the remaining part of the breathing session. However, after 10 min of practice you realized that you can have 12 seconds exhalations with no problems at all. Then you can finish the session with slightly longer exhalations and BCD. Your new or final BCD will be 16 seconds.

Note 2. If during the later part of the session, not after first 2-3 minutes, you find that you cannot continue with the same BCD, you should take rest and stop the session. For example, imagine that you started the session with 2 seconds in and 7 seconds out. You could maintain this breath pattern for more than 5 minutes. However, after 7 min you felt too tired and breathless. Then you should take rest and think about the possible causes of your low adaptation reserves (why your organism cannot experience positive adaptation to this breathing exercise. Possible causes include: nutritional deficiencies (EFA, Ca, Mg, Zn, K, Na, etc.); chronic sleep deprivation or insufficient deep sleep; lack of cortisol, or thyroxin or some other hormones in the body; etc.)

Your success, apart from all preliminary parameters, depends on the following factors:

- comfortable maximum inhalations using your diaphragm only, while keeping chest muscles relaxed;

- slow long and maximum exhalations (exhale even more than you do during your usual exhalation);

- relaxation of all body muscles especially during exhalations.

8.5 Duration of one breathing session

A lasting positive change in breathing of adults is achieved after 10-12 minutes of practice. The CP gets higher for the next 4-10 hours depending on the influence of life-style factors later. However, a good session can be about 15-20 min long so that you feel and experience more energy, better focus, sharper mind, improved logic and other encouraging and positive effects after the session.

The suggested durations of breathing sessions for children are:

5-10 years old – 2 breathing sessions per day 7-10 min each or 3 sessions 5-7 min each;

11-15 years old – 2 breathing sessions per day 10-15 min each or 3 sessions 7-10 min each.

8.6 Typical symptoms during the breathing session

It is normal to experience:

- warm extremities (hands and feet) or even heat in the whole body (increased CO_2 in body cells);

- increased salivation due to stimulations of glands of the GI tract since mucosal surfaces are under gentle massage created by periodic alterations in air pressure (from negative to positive).

8.7 Measure and record your parameters after the session

When you finish the session measure your final heart rate during 30 seconds and write it down in your daily log. About 2-3 minutes later measure your final CP and write it down as well. Compare these final numbers with initial ones.

In addition, listen to your breathing for about 20-30 seconds so that to compare your new breathing pattern after the session with the breathing pattern that you had before the session. This will help you to have better understanding of what does it mean to achieve changes in your usual or basal breathing and to understand the reduced breathing exercises, which you may learn later.

8.8 Criteria of success

There are 3 main criteria indicating good adaptation of your organism to a breathing session.

1. During the session you should feel warmer, especially in your hands and feet. (This sign is present in most, but not all people.)

2. Immediately after you finish the session or 5-10 minutes later, your final heart rate should be slower.

3. Your final CP should be higher.

Statistically, after the correct 15-20 min breathing session, the heart rate decreases by about 2-4 beats per minute and the CP increases by 3-7 seconds at least. Your higher CP is the main sign of your lighter breathing and better body oxygenation.

Be aware that your heart rate can be higher immediately after the session. If it so, measure it again in 10 minutes. It may remain high if you recently consumed caffeine (coffee, strong tea, chocolate, etc.). I do not discourage, for example, drinking coffee since it helps people with low CPs to be more alert and function better throughout the day. (Keep in mind that at higher CPs, about 35-40 seconds and especially at even larger numbers, coffee and other products with caffeine are going to produce unpleasant effects: nervousness, anxiety, racing heart, etc.)

8.9 If there is no progress

Over 97% of students are able to achieve the above-mentioned positive changes from their first attempts, if they follow the above-mentioned suggestions. If you feel worse after the session (dizziness, lightheadedness, etc.), then usually all 3 criteria will yield negative results as well: your extremities will not be warmer, your final heart rate will be higher, and your final CP will be less. How to deal with this rare problem? Make an easier DIY device:

1. Use wider tube

2. Use shorter tube

3. Reduce the volume of the plastic bottle part.

In addition, make your next breathing session easier: breathe more comfortably and/or exhale faster and do not try to create air hunger. Breathe freely and without any air hunger for the first 2-3 minutes and then gradually extend your exhalations. Again, record your CP and pulse changes. Analyze your results after the session in relation to 3 criteria of success. If there is an improvement, practice this easier version of breathing exercises for 1 week at least. When your CP is higher, you can try a more difficult breathing device and more challenging types of the breathing exercise.

There are very rare cases, when a person still has difficulties with improving their main physiological parameters (the CP and pulse). If this is the case with you, introduce further modification for the next breathing session: inhale air through the nose and exhale through the device comfortably. Continue to breathe in this manner: in through the nose, out through the device. Measure your parameters after the

102

session. Here again, you should achieve some improvement in your state of health before trying more difficult exercise versions.

If you still cannot achieve positive effects in more than one third of your breathing sessions, these breathing sessions are not useful for your current health state. You should not continue these sessions until you find the cause of your problems. Among possible causes are: loss of CO_2 sensitivity, cortisol deficiency, thyroxin deficiency, severe EFA or Ca deficiency, lack or absence of deep stages of sleep, constant allergic reactions, etc. If you cannot find the answer, you will require special attention from an experienced breathing teacher.

You should also stop the session, if you experience breathlessness and fatigue during the session with a drop in your BCD, as we discussed above.

8.10 Which time of the day is best for breathing sessions?

It depends mainly on your daily CP changes and other personal factors. For most people, the best time to practice the breathing session is after your last large meal is digested or at about 9-10 pm before going to bed. This will help you to get higher MCP (morning control pause). However, breathing sessions can be practiced at other times providing you follow the suggestions explained in this manual.

8.11 Can a session be practiced in the morning after waking up?

If your MCP (morning CP) is much less than your usual daily numbers, you should correct life style factors related to sleep (download corresponding manuals from the website www.NormalBreathing.com) and you can have a breathing session after waking up before breakfast. However, if your MCP is about the same as usual daily numbers, you should start the day with some physical exercise. Afterwards you can have 1 session in the morning and/or other breathing sessions during the day, including one session before sleep.

8.12 Total duration of daily breath-work

The more you practice, the faster your weekly CP growth. If one practices for about 40 min per day, for most people, their CP growth can be as high as 3-5 seconds or even more. (The main factors that make our health restoration slow are: obesity, amount of previously taken medications, age and lack of physical exercise.)

However, even if you practice for only 20 minutes per day, you still should be able to gradually get higher CP numbers, but only with about 1-2 seconds morning CP increase in 1 week. For this light version of breathing retraining, in order to move forward, you should focus on life-style factors.

The total suggested durations of daily breathing sessions for children:

5-10 years old – 15-20 minutes per day;

11-15 years old – 20-30 minutes per day.

8.13 Morning CP growth

Many students ask the following question. *Why does my MCP not increase steadily, day after day?* Indeed, when a student analyzes their progress, they notice that their MCP does not increase steadily day after day. This may become a discouraging factor. However, temporary CP drops, for 1-3 days, are normal.

You should persist with exercises since the MCP will recover later to even larger numbers. Hence, you should evaluate your average MCP increase by analyzing your daily log for a whole week.

Another common question is: *How much is a typical weekly MCP increase?*

It is usual that the MCP increases by about 2-5 seconds every week (until about 35 seconds MCP), if the person has 30-40 min for breathing exercises and about 1-1.5 hour for physical exercise every day with strictly nasal breathing. However, there are 3 main factors that influence one's rate of progress:

1) **Obesity** (it is more difficult for obese people to progress);

2) **Age** (it is slightly more difficult for older people to increase their MCP);

3) **Amount of total medication consumed and duration of their diseases**.

Hence, a typical sick person has about 15 seconds usual daily CP and about 10-12 seconds for the MCP. Hence, it takes about 2-4 weeks for a person with mild asthma, bronchitis, heart disease, CFS, etc. to achieve over a 20 second CP 24/7.

8.14 Will I progress steadily up to 2-3 min MCP all the time?

For higher CPs, your maximum achievement mainly depends on the amount of time that you devote to physical and breathing exercises. If you spend about 2 hours on rigorous physical exercise and about 1 hour on breathing exercises, potentially you may almost constantly progress up to 2-3 min MCP. However, such situations are very rare.

First, most people spend only about 1.5-2 hours in total for breathing exercises and physical activity. Hence, they can achieve only about 25-30 seconds for MCP. (Note that many of these people were ruled by symptoms and medication for many years and these CPs are experienced as a profound shift to better health.)

Second, those people, who devote up to 3 hours to their health, usually get stuck with about 35 seconds MCP, often for many weeks or months before breaking through to 40 seconds MCP (so that one's MCP becomes more than 40 s) is the hardest CP threshold during breathing retraining. Note that 35 seconds MCP is a great achievement that results in shorter sleep (naturally) and many other effects described elsewhere.

However, to break through 40 seconds MCP requires some additional methods and techniques which are described in other manuals and books. I teach it separately as a Level 3 ("Normal health") course, but there are some students who manage to get through 40 seconds MCP based on information that is provided during the common Level 2 ("Existence") course.

8.15 Why is a daily log necessary?

Our goal is to change our unconscious breathing pattern so that one has more oxygen in the cells of the organism after the session. Hence, the person gradually raises their CP, slows their breathing, and obtains a lower heart rate at rest. We target long-term changes in our basal (or unconscious) breathing. Your progress will be faster, if you are able to identify and address 2-3 of the most important life-style factors that slow down your progress. Hence, you should develop your detective skills. Since all these changes in your health are slow (they require days or even weeks), it is impossible to keep all the related information in mind (all breathing sessions, your medication, symptoms, meals, sleep, supplements, etc. for the whole period of time).

Changes in breathing are often difficult to notice. For example, many people do not feel much worse when they slouch or become slightly overheated. The CP can easily drop by 5 or even more seconds and the person will notice nothing. In fact, due to increased excitability of the brain, we often invent pleasant myths and fantasies and may feel even better due to avoidance of the real world. This is one of the reasons why hyperventilation can go unnoticed or even get perceived positively by our minds. However, when we have solid numbers (especially, the CP and heart rate), we have a more clear picture about our real physiological and spiritual state. Hence, it is useful to record everything that matters in your daily log.

The Appendix of this book has the daily log. It can be used for both types of breathing sessions: using the DIY breathing device and Buteyko breathing exercises. You can copy this page or download the daily log (Word or PDF file) from the "Downloads" section of www.NormalBreathing.com: http://www.normalbreathing.com/free-downloads.php.

8.16 How to fill your daily log

Here is a part of a personal daily log with numbers related to 3 breathing sessions (3 rows or 3 lines). Each line of the daily log corresponds to one breathing session.

Date	MCP	Time (hour)	Init. pulse	Init CP	Breath cycle and session time	Final pulse	Final CP	PE, min	Symptoms, medication and auxiliary activities
7.04	11 s	10 am	78	15	20 s; 15 min	74	21	30	1 puff of ventolin
		9 pm	74	20	22 s; 20 min	72	28		10 ml fish oil
8.04	14 s	7 am	76	19	23 s; 20 min	74	24	50	no ventolin

On April 7, the person had 11 seconds for MCP (Morning Control Pause). He took one puff of ventolin (see the last column). At 10 am he did the first breathing session. His initial heart rate was 78 beats per min (heart rate is measured during 30 seconds time period). His initial CP was 15 seconds. The breathing session had 20 seconds for the BCD (breathing cycle duration). Have a clock to count it. The session lasted for 15 minutes.

His final pulse (after he finished the morning breathing session) was 74 beats per minute and his CP 21 seconds. He had 30 min of physical exercise for this day.

The last column is for information about your symptoms, medication, supplements, special activities (e.g., travels, sleeping in other places, taping mouth at night, use of belts at night), changes in diet, and anything else that can influence your breathing and general health.

9. Breathing retraining program

Your general progress depends mainly on your persistence, self-discipline, right breathing exercises, and ability to figure out and correct those life style factors which are particularly destructive for your body oxygenation and general health. If you have consistent improvements in your wellbeing, pulse and the CP, you are on the right track. Congratulations!

9.1 More challenging breathing exercises

Some students like challenges and even try to create conditions for more difficult breathing sessions. You can do so, if your body positively accepts the previous breathing sessions. What can be suggested? After 3-4 days of breathing exercises in a comfortable regime, if the main parameters (the heart rate and CP) are improved after all or almost all breathing sessions, such students can proceed to more intensive types of breathing sessions by creating more resistance during inhalations and exhalations and/or increasing the volume of the bottle part (so that to get more CO_2 back in the lungs and other parts and organs of your body).

Warning. If you have any above-mentioned diseases or conditions (transplanted organs; heart disease; panic attacks; asthma, COPD, or other problems with lungs; type 2 diabetes; pregnancy; etc.), you should apply the rules outlined for these specific situations.

More challenging breathing exercise or devices can be made using various techniques:

1. You can squeeze or bend a part of the vinyl tube with your fingers for more resistance especially during inhalations.

2. Make a combined device by adding a very short piece of narrower tube (only about 3-6 mm in inner diameter and 3-10 cm long) to your original device. Insert this additional tube (extension) into the

free end of your original tube and try this combined device for 2-3 minutes. (These tubes are often sold in stores with the expectation that a next narrower tube will fit inside the previous larger tube as it is shown on right.)

3. You can make a breathing device with a longer and/or narrower tube.

4. You can increase the volume of air on the plastic bottle part. Use another plastic bottle with larger volume left (up to 500-700 ml for 20-25 second CP students and up to 1 L or more for 30 second CP students).

As a result of these innovations, if your current CP is about 25 seconds or more, you can create such a device so that your inhalation, even with all your efforts, can be about 9-11 seconds at least. Then you have to apply mild effort for exhalations as well. Occasionally, such breathing sessions can make students sweat, but again, if there is a positive response from the body, your health will get better even if you perspire.

You may buy and try a more narrow tube (e.g., 4 mm inner diameter). If you manage to breathe through it for only 3-5 minutes, you should be able to go on for longer time (up to 15-20 min or more) and it would be the most efficient breathing session for you.

If you find the narrow tube impossible (you cannot breathe through it, even when trying to breathe hard in- and-out, for more than 1-2 minutes), there are 3 options to make the device easier:

1) You can reduce the volume of the bottle by trimming its bottom part using scissors;

2) You can make the length of the tube shorter;

3) You can use a wide tube for a while.

Later, when your CP is higher, you will be able to use the narrower tube.

9.2 Breath work and life style factors for over 20 second CP 24/7

While breathing exercises are targeted to lighten your breathing for several hours after each session, it is important to maintain positive changes by addressing abnormal life styles and other factors that make your breathing heavier. Consider a following typical example. A student can practice the best breathing exercises, but if their CP significantly drops during night sleep, especially due to sleeping on their back and breathing through the mouth at night causing allergic inflammation in sinuses or airways, then this student will never get more than 20 seconds morning CP and never recover from their main health problems.

Since for over 97% students the CP is an accurate predictor of the current health state, getting over 20 second CP 24/7 is the step that allows to achieve stability and to stop progression of most serious chronic conditions.

What are the required steps or conditions for over 20 second CP 24/7?

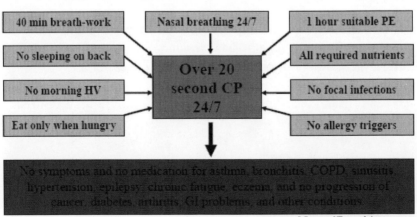

www.NormalBreathing.com

Explanations and notes.

Very few people require additional hormonal support (cortisol, thyroxin, etc.) in order to get over 20 second CP.

Sometimes, it is necessary to temporarily interrupt some activities that involve hours of hyperventilation. For example, if a person sings or speaks (lectures) every day for 5 or more hours, then these periods of overbreathing may prevent the person from getting over 20 seconds MCP. Such people often require a temporary break to focus on their health. Later, when they get over 20 or more second CP 24/7, they can resume their favorite or desired activities with greatly improved quality.

Let us consider these factors in more detail.

A 40 min breath-work can be 2 breathing sessions each 20 min long, or 3 sessions about 13-14 min long, or 4 sessions at 10 min each.

Among other most fundamental steps are **Prevention of breathing through the mouth** and **Prevention of sleeping on one's back**. There are 2 manuals that can be used, if relevant: Manual "How to prevent sleeping on one's back" Manual "How to maintain nasal breathing 24/7". They are both provided in the last part (Appendixes) of this book.

No morning HV means no morning hyperventilation (i.e., the CP drop throughout the night should be no more than 5 seconds, preferably less than 3 s). Hence, you have to solve all problems that cause your overnight CP drop.

1 hour suitable PE means 1 hour of total Physical Exercise every day with strictly nasal breathing (in and out) all the time. Usually, less than 20 seconds current CP means feeling tired and inability to do running, jogging, or any other rigorous exercise with strictly nasal breathing for most people. However, walking is possible. Moreover, with further CP increase, students feel empowered and surprised by energy and skills previously hidden in their sick bodies. The initial requirement for physical exercise is to have at least 1 hour every day in total.

All required nutrients are partially considered in the big book "Normal breathing: the key to vital health" and in the manual "Your guide to nutrients that improve breathing and body oxygenation" (to be available soon). The most common deficiencies include fish oil, calcium, magnesium, zinc, and protein. Some other nutritional deficiencies can also slow down or even halt breathing retraining. Mild cortisol deficiency can also be corrected using a special nutritional support described in the manual.

"Eat only when hungry" is the central common sense rule developed by Dr. Buteyko in relation to meals. It also means that you should stop eating at first signs of satiety.

Note for overweight and obese people. If you are overweight and crave or eager to eat fats (except fish oil) or starchy foods (bread, rice, potatoes, etc), you are hyperventilating. Instead of eating, do another breathing session to normalize your blood glucose level and reduce your hunger pangs. If you eat any calorie-rich foods, your CP will get further down. Your progress will be linked to your weight loss. Breathing exercises naturally rise blood glucose levels so that you can feel no hunger for calorie-rich foods.

You can surely enjoy all other foods, like vegetables, greens, some fruits, lean meat, fat-free dairy, beans and lentils, etc., if they are a part of your usual diet.

No focal infections requires your analysis or certain health conditions which can not be solved using breathing retraining only. For example, if you have large intestinal parasites, depending on the toxic load, your current CP will be restricted by 25-35 seconds or even smaller numbers. There are 4 focal infections:

1. **Large intestinal parasites** (roundworms, flatworms, hookworms, liver flukes, etc.)

2. **Dental cavities** (caries or pathogenic anaerobes in teeth)

3. **Dead tonsils** (degenerated tonsils that do not have blood supply and harbor pathogenic bacteria)

4. **Feet mycosis** (or athlete's foot).

Sometimes, presence of root canals or mercury amalgams can become the main issue that requires radical solution for higher CP. All these challenges are explained in detail in the manual "Breathing retraining and focal infections" (to be available soon).

No allergy triggers involves avoidance of any triggers of your allergic responses. These triggers may include:
- air-born dust mites, cat and dog proteins, mold, pollen, paper ink, chemicals, pollutants, and fumes;
- digested gluten products, dairy products, peanuts, tomatoes, and many other foods and substances;
- tap water or other consumed liquids with chemical triggers present;
- substances and objects that can produce an allergic response due to skin contact (synthetic clothes, detergents, paints, metals, plastics, etc.);
- electromagnetic and other penetrating radiation.

Regular allergic inflammatory response exhausts cortisol reserves and suppresses the immune system making breathing normalization very difficult or even impossible.

There are many other life-style factors that can significantly influence one's CP progress. For example, prolonged sun-bathing (up to 30 min or more) causes most humans to hyperventilate lowering their CP. Taking a cold shower, on the other hand, is great for helping to achieve normalization of your breathing. There are, however, several necessary safety rules to follow. The most important one is over 20 second CP. (More details can be found in my article "Who and when can safely take cold shower").

9.3 Future progress

While getting over 20 seconds for one's MCP (morning CP) is a great first step towards better health and elimination of major symptoms for many health conditions, the real health starts ar over 50 s CP. Why is it necessary or desirable to get over 50 s MCP? Well, the life with less than 40 s MCP is a struggle. This means that, for example, exercise for most people is not fun and joy even when they have about 35 s MCP. (Of course, there are exceptions.) Natural sleep is too long (it is usually about 6-6.5 hours for 35 s MCP), and level of energy is not high. People do not enjoy raw food and often like to eat junk food. There are many other lifestyle choices indicating poor health.

Here is the Table that reflects some of changes in their **natural choices** that people make in relation to their lifestyle. Each person whom I taught and knew could tell that these changes are true.

Lifestyle factor:	Body oxygen < 30 s	Body oxygen > 50 s
Energy level	Medium, low, or very low	High
Desire to exercise	Not strong, but possible	Craving and joy of exercise
Intensive exercise with nose breathing	Hard or impossible	Easy and effortless
Typical mind states	Confusion, anxiety, depression	Focus, concentration, clarity
Craving for coffee, sugar and junk foods	Present	Absent
Addictions to smoking, alcohol, and drugs	Possible	Absent
Desire to eat raw foods	Weak and rare	Very common and natural
Correct posture	Rare and requires efforts	Natural and automatic
Sleep	Often of poor quality; > 7 hours	Excellent quality; < 5 hours naturally

However, nearly each Buteyko breathing doctor in Russia and breathing practitioner on the West can confirm that it is the most difficult challenge in breathing retraining to break through 40 s morning CP. The most common scenario is that diligent students can get even up to 50-60 seconds for their daily CP numbers, but their morning CP is about 33-35 seconds. Such pattern can be present for weeks, months or even years.

While there are many factors that are crucial for breaking through 40 s morning CP (so that you have more than 40 seconds for several mornings in row), physical exercise, according to Dr. Buteyko, is the main factor that defines the long-term success of the student. It is particularly beneficial, when it is accompanied by perspiration (sweating) and prolonged shaking (mechanical vibrations of the body), as it takes place during jogging. Since lack of physical exercise is the main cause of hyperventilation in modern man, it is normal that daily duration of physical activity has a correlation with personal morning CP. Indeed, Buteyko and his colleagues found that when their students achieved high CPs (e.g., up to 60 s) and stopped doing breathing exercises, the CPs of these students will depend on the amount of daily physical exercise, even in cases, when these students continued to control their breath, while involved in other activities.

Below is a table that is based on writings of Dr. K. Buteyko and my own observations of students. This table established a link between the duration of daily physical activity and maximum expected MCP for experienced students. (Note that in order to recover from chronic diseases, one generally require more physical exercise than suggested here).

Duration of physical exercise per day	Maximum body O2 expected
0 min	15 s
30 min	20 s
60 min	25 s
1 hour of devoted PE + 1 hour others	30 s
1.5 hour of devoted PE + 1 hour others	35 s
2 hours of devoted PE + 1 hour others	Up to 2-3 min

Table note. "1.5 hour of devoted PE + 1 hour others" means that the person spends, for example, 1.5 hour for devoted PE (physical exercise) (e.g., 2 daily jogging sessions 45 min each) and also gets 1 hour of walking here and there throughout the day.

Many sick people, especially city dwellers, often have less than 20 min of physical exercise per day. (These 20 minutes include walking within the house, to the car, while shopping, etc.). Their MCP is, at best, according to this table, less than 20 seconds.

If a person with over 20 second CP devotes 1 hour to rigorous physical exercise with strictly nasal breathing, they can finally get stabilized, over a period of some days, at the level of 25 seconds MCP. Usually such people also naturally get about 30 min of light exercise throughout the day (e.g., walking here and there).

Having more than 2 hours of daily physical exercise is generally sufficient to get or maintain any CP.

Elderly people often require less physical exercise than suggested by the Table above, while teenagers and young people in their 20s and 30s sometimes may require more physical activity to achieve the CP numbers provided by the Table. Other factors, including diet, chewing, supplements, daily work, and sleep conditions, also influence the achieved CP level.

When starting the program of breathing retraining, students generally progress steadily up to about 35 seconds MCP, if they get daily sufficient physical exercise. After achieving 35 seconds MCP most students can get stuck there for weeks or months. To break through the 40 seconds MCP (so that the student has over 40 seconds for the MCP) is the most difficult challenge in breathing retraining. Some people are able to progress smoothly up to 40-50 daily CPs, while using the above-described tools. However, most students require a special program and explanation of details specific for this challenge (how to break through 40 s MCP). Practice shows that for further progress (up to 60 s CP and more), it is necessary to learn the reduced breathing exercises developed by Dr. Konstantin Buteyko.

The advantage of the Buteyko exercises is that they can be practiced anywhere without devices. At higher CPs and after some weeks or months of practice, many students become motivated and capable of practicing reduced breathing exercises for many hours every day, while being involved in other activities and without any detrimental effects on the quality of these other activities (reading, watching TV, driving, walking, etc.).

You may find a Buteyko breathing teacher who can explain to you how to practice Buteyko breathing exercises or, if your CP is about 30 s or more, you can learn these exercises, for example, from the big book "Normal Breathing: the Key to Vital Health".

I plan to write a separate book that provides essential details and important practical suggestions that explain how to break trough 40 s morning CP and start to enjoy real physical health.

9.4 Final remarks

Feel free to send your comments and observations about this manual, as well as your success story (personal testimonial) so that it can be shared with others to encourage them to try breathing retraining and regain vital health. If you require my further help or personal consultations you can also contact me: artour_rakhimov (at) hotmail.com.

Success and easy breathing, Artour Rakhimov

www.NormalBreathing.com

10 Testimonials of people who tried the DIY breathing device

10.1 Asthma (chronic and severe cases)

From: Steve, 46

I was an asthmatic for over 30 years since my early teens. In my late teens, I gained about 40 pounds and got all kinds of awful health problems. I was on two different inhalers (10-15 times a day) and nebulizers (1-2 a day). I was in the emergency room every month. During each trip I felt miserable and disgusting there. When I found Buteyko, my CP was 8 seconds. I started to practice breathing exercises with my own DIY device 3 times per day and my morning CP went up to about 25 s after 4 weeks. I was truly amazed. Now I'm in control of my personal health again: no medication at all. I am not reacting to triggers like mold, dust mites or other airborne irritants anymore. Even if you had asthma for decades, the Buteyko therapy can make a big difference! All my symptoms are gone... I breathe shallowly through my nose, and that has been the foundation of my success. Thank you, Artour, for your care about simple people.

From: Margaret, 58

I've had asthma since infancy..... Solution? It involves breathing exercises practiced diligently until the body learns to breathe normally. This program (www.normalbreathing.com) with the DIY breathing device is phenomenal. I have not used my puffer once since starting a month ago, compared with 15-20 puffs a day prior. My initial CP was about 9 s! In 3 weeks I was getting up to 25-30 s of oxygen in the body... Every day I go for a 7 km walk and not once have I feel tired or short of breath. In fact I felt strong and could have kept going. Every other time I have needed to stop for breath and use the puffer. The secret was/is the nose breathing. Close the mouth and breathe exclusively through the nose, even when you exercise. It is a miracle in my life. I am very thankful to you Artour for this manual.

From: Ahmed Hussein, 45

I am 45 years old and have been an asthmatic virtually all my life. I have had sinus problems most of my life. I had my first asthma attack at the age of 28 and was in the hospital for 5 days after coming close to death. My breathing stayed very heavy since then: I'd be winded walking from my bed to the bathroom in the morning. My drugs were at about $1,000 dollars a month for years... I found the DIY breathing retraining manual on the internet and after the second day of intensive breathing retraining, my sinuses cleared, the tightness in my chest disappeared, my lungs cleared and the secretions stopped. In addition I felt more relaxed, alert and generally well. I have been off all drugs in 2 weeks. My CP tripled since I started the breathing exercises and I am determined to get up to 60 s CP. Please, let me express here my gratitude for your help.

From: Greg Neil, 34

I had extremely bad asthma: using a ventolin inhaler very frequently and taking becloforte (corticosteroid, 6 puffs 3 times a day); uniphyllin tablets (twice a day); and prednisolone tablets (another corticosteroid, 10 to 20 mgs a day depending on my state). I was hospitalized a few times, including two times in an ER: oxymeter reading of 40, steroids and about 8 nebulizers in the ER alone with my pulse over 160. When I started Buteyko and DIY device exercises I had less than 10 s CP. I hated the idea of taping up my mouth but tried it. Now I tape up each night! It makes a huge difference in the morning. By the end of the first week, I stopped using ventolin and uniphyllin completely. In 3 weeks I have cut down all my medication, but my morning CP is still only about 18 s. The Buteyko method does require conscious awareness of our breathing for a year or more. Even if it takes longer than this to breathe shallowly automatically I will continue to apply the method and practice exercises with my breathing device as it has made such a huge difference to my asthma.

10.2 Bronchitis

From: Mike, 26

The breathing course has significantly changed my life. For over 3 years I was being treated for chronic bronchitis. I was getting more and more of steroids, antibiotics, and bronchodilators. Then I decided to try Buteyko breathing retraining using the DIY breathing device. Just after 1 month of breathing exercises with the DIY breathing device, I have had no bronchitis and no medication at all. I can easily go running now for 40 minutes with breathing only through the nose. My sleep and energy level are about 10 times better. I wish to thank you again for your sincere concern for helping us to overcome our various illnesses.

From: Cicilia, 47

I was panting at the slightest exertion, even from walking 50 m or climbing as few as 10 stairs. Since starting my breathing sessions (November 2009) I am now off all medication. This winter (2010) I have had no colds, flu or bronchitis. My immune system and general health has dramatically improved, all thanks to you Artour and to Buteyko.

From: Dorothy, 31

For 2 years I was desperate. I had severe chronic bronchitis. Winters were horrible: one bout of pneumonia or bronchitis after the other. My health was worsening month after month. One day I came across the Buteyko method on the internet. Then I downloaded the manual "Amazing DIY breathing device" from Artour. Within 3 weeks I reduced my medication to one puff in the morning. My general health has improved dramatically. I have not had a single infection after starting the Buteyko method. Thanks to you for committing your time to teach this valuable information.

10.3 Emphysema

From: Susan, 56

I only had 25% of my lungs left when I begun using the DIY water device I'm getting a lot better. Before starting this work, I was on a nebulizer machine every three hours 24/7 and that means I was up every three hours at night also and sometimes every hour. I was on every inhaler you can imagine. My doctors told me there was nothing else they could do for me. I was at the emergency room three times a week and in the hospital once a month sometimes for a week at a time and sometimes two weeks at a time. Today, it has been almost 3 years since I've used the DIY device. I started with a miserable 7 s CP. My lungs are now over 60% now and I can go days without using the nebulizer machine. If I have to use it, I will use it only once instead of 15 or 20 a day. For the first time in twelve years I'm beginning to have a life and hope, and it is all because of Buteyko. My morning CP is now about 25 s. I can take long walks now! I practice for 60 min every day (3 breathing sessions for 20 min with the DIY device) and will continue doing so. Thank you, Artour, for all your great work in writing and sharing this invaluable knowledge.

From: Arnold, 51

I suffered from sleep apnea for over 10 years and emphysema for 3 years. It got so bad that I was hospitalized 4 times to an emergency room. I was so breathless that I literally could do nothing more then lie on the couch while waiting for my wife to find me. I began the use of bronchodilators and steroids, as well as 24 hour O2 therapy. Once browsing the net, I downloaded the manual about breathing retraining and the DIY device. I re-read it 4 times. Within three days after getting the manual - I stopped bronchodilators and put aside the oxygen tanks. It has been hard but it works! In 5 months of practice I feel better than I have felt in 7 years. What are the changes? My sinuses are clear, no wheezing, no coughing; I have lost over 20 pounds, my sleep is great …

From: Mike, 68

I had emphysema and snoring with horrible mornings and foggy head. I used to wake 3-4 times in a night with very dry mouth and need to get up to drink water. My medications before the Buteyko course: Pulmicort, Prednisone, Atrovent, Rani, etc. After one month of breathing through my favorite toy (the DIY device), I cut all medication except 2 puffs of Pulmicort per day. My sleep is now perfect. Now I am waking up in the morning with a clearer head (thanks to mouth taping and higher MCP) and have also stopped snoring. I will persist until I get my lungs normal and my CP is up to 60 s or more. It is very important to do breathing exercises daily and follow all other ideas related to life style factors. Each of them (nasal breathing only, sleeping on the left side or chest, eating only when really hungry, proper nutrients, etc.) are crucial for success. Many thanks for all your help.

10.4 Multiple chemical sensitivities

From: Anna, 51

I used to get a stuffy nose very easily and had multiple chemical sensitivities. My sense of smell was increased and I was highly sensitive to semi-strong scents like cigarettes, perfume, and paint. I got tightness in my chest every once in a while and upon regular exercise got easily winded. I noticed that upon starting breathing exercises, my nose cleared up within days. The biggest problem that existed for about five years before the course was an allergy-like reaction to cigarette smoke. This problem decreased after a week of the breathing exercises. It used to be that I had to run from the smell if I was anywhere near a lit up cigarette. Now I can even be in the same car with someone smoking, and not have to worry because I react like a regular person. You have no idea how that makes me feel after years of suffering and feeling like an outcast due to it. There's no way I will ever go back to the way I used to breathe. My morning CP is about 32 seconds. I am able to breathe normally around smoke without feeling sick for the first time in five years.

10.5 Chronic fatigue syndrome

From: Andrea, 27

I used to suffer from Chronic Fatigue Syndrome. Since 2004 I had to stay in bed for weeks feeling totally exhausted. I was so tired, I could hardly move my body parts. Two weeks after starting the breathing retraining my chronic fatigue is gone. My initial CP was 6 seconds. By the end of the first week I had build it up to 20 seconds. Now it is in the mid thirties. I am much more calm and relaxed. My cravings for coffee and sugar are gone. I am a different person. I am in control of my health and life.

From: Ron, 59

My chronic fatigue started about 15 years ago. For the first 4 years my health was getting progressively worse. Previously, I enjoyed daily runs, up to 15-25 km per day for about 2 decades. After getting sick, my physical fitness was greatly reduced. When I tried light jogging for 20-40 min only (it was too hard to run more) in cold weather, I would get sick with infections for the next 2-3 days: fever (over 38 degrees), a very soar throat, a husky voice, a totally blocked nose and a lot of mucus. My sleep was up to 11-12 hours per night and it was horrible: waking up several times every night, tossing in the bed for 30-60 min or more, and I also had headaches... My first CP measurement was 7 seconds. In 1 week of breathing retraining I was up to 20 s. In 2 months, I was up to 50-60 s of oxygen in the morning. My my sleep is down to 4 hours now: I fall asleep in about 1 minute and wake up in what feels like a moment later only to find out that 4 hours passed in a flash. After my sleep, I am again full of energy and have no desire to sleep more. I haven't had a single infection after I started my breath retraining. What is even more surprising is that when I got over 40 s MCP, I started to crave physical activity. I do not run, I virtually fly above ground with ... light nasal breathing. I go running for 1.5-2 hours every day and feel even stronger than I was 20 years ago! It is the most incredible health therapy I ever tried and experienced.

10.6 Sinusitis or nasal congestion

From: Bret, 23

I had problems with sinuses for many years. My nose was totally blocked all the time. I lost all sense of smell. My initial CP was about 9 s. After finding out about Buteyko and his method, I got a manual and made my personal DIY breathing device. In a week I was able to breath through my nose most of the time. In less than a month I achieved over 20 s CP 24/7. I can now sense different smells and aromas and my nose is clear. I should thank Dr. Buteyko and you, Artour for this amazing method.

10.7 Hypertension

From: Otto, 63

After three weeks of the DIY device practice my blood pressure went down to a normal level and it has stayed there ever since. My sleep and digestion have improved, I breathe easier and I can even run 5 km without feeling tired. It has been the most amazing change in my health and life! Thank you for your great work.

10.8 Hypertension and anxiety

From: Mary, 45

Thanks to breathing exercises I learned how to control panic attacks (when I feel that they are approaching) and keep my blood pressure normal. I do not take any blood pressure medication anymore. My CP increased from about 12 to 30 s. Another of the benefits of the breathing exercises is that I sleep really well, only for 6 hours, and wake up feeling refreshed. In the past, 9 hours of sleep were not enough. I plan to increase my physical activity up to 1.5-2 hours per day and get an even higher CP.

10.9 Chronic cough

From: Huan, 27

I got problems with chronic coughing after severe carbon monoxide poisoning. On top of that weeks later I developed various digestive problems (bloating, irritable bowel, GERD, etc.). For over 3 years I tried almost everything: supplements, herbs, fasting, colonic irrigation, acupuncture, etc. Some of these things could improve by symptoms but only for a few days. While searching the internet, I stumbled over Buteyko, but I dismissed it. Finally, out of desperation, I tried the breathing retraining program from the DIY-device manual written by Artour (www. Normalbreathing.com) and within the first 3 days I started to sleep much better and my cough bouts become about 4-5 times shorter in duration. Eventually, when my CP got up to 30 s, all coughing has stopped. I have even more energy now than prior to Buteyko. Thank you, Artour, for your wonderful work.

From: Michelle, 29

My 9-year son developed a chronic hacking cough at 7. His mouth and throat were always full of mucus and required clearing. For two years we were going from one specialist to another (respirologist, ear-nose-throat, allergy) and they could not find the cause. None of the drugs they suggested and we tried worked. After practicing the breathing exercises ("Amazing DIY Breathing Device") for just one month, his cough is absolutely gone!

11 Appendix

11. 1 How to maintain nasal breathing during the day

Breathing through the mouth is a sign of chronic hyperventilation. Healthy people (over 40 or 60 s CP) do not breathe through the mouth at all. If they try, their CP will be below 40 s. On the other hand, if you observe sick people, you will notice that breathing through the mouth is their frequent characteristic.

The very first step, in order to solve this problem, is education so that you completely realize importance of nasal breathing 24/7. Hence, importance of educational pages of this website.

The second step is your irrevocable decision to breathe through the nose all the time when you are awake. Any time when your nose gets blocked, you should apply Module 4-B (The Emergency Procedure for blocked nose). You can do it 10, 20, or 50 times per day.

If you find that your mouth is dry in the morning, consider the following experience of Dr. Buteyko's patients. In order to ensure nasal breathing during the night, in the 1960s Russian patients invented mouth taping. First of all, it is necessary to find out if one has this problem by checking dryness in the mouth just after waking up in the morning. If the mouth is dry, the person had mouth breathing. It could begin when the person went to sleep or it could appear at 3 or 4 am. In any case, just 20-30 min of mouth-breathing resets the breathing centre to lower CPs, and such patients, as a ruler, have less than 20 s CP in the morning. Moreover, if you have a malignant tumor and your daily CP is above 20 s, your tumor will grow only during the time of the night, when you breathe through your mouth. If you have sinusitis, the pathogenic bacteria in your sinuses will multiply and colonize new mucosal surfaces when you breathe through your mouth.

Organic damage to the heart muscle, growth of inflamed areas in the GI tract, advance of pathogens on your skin (in cases of eczema, psoriasis, etc.), and many other problems will appear if your mouth gets open during your sleep. Solution? You need to tape your mouth.

11.2 How to tape one's mouth at night to prevent mouth breathing during sleep

For mouth taping one needs a surgical tape and cream to prevent the tape sticking. Both can be bought in the pharmacy. Micropore (or 3M) and vaselin are popular choices. First, put a small amount of cream on the lips so that it is easy to remove the tape in the morning. Then take a small piece of tape and stick it in the middle, vertically, across the closed mouth. Some students prefer to put it along or horizontally, but a small piece in the middle is sufficient. If you are afraid to "seal" your mouth completely, tape only one half of the mouth leaving space for emergency breathing.

In 2006 one of my Buteyko colleagues, Dr. James Oliver, a GP from the UK and former president of the Buteyko Breathing Association made a presentation to the British Thoracic Society about the safety of mouth taping based on thousands of cases both in Russia and in the west. Previously he conducted a survey among us, Buteyko teachers and obtained the statistical data.

Taping at night normally should be a temporary measure. When one's CP is above 20 s in the morning, mouth taping is not necessary.

Can mouth taping create distress?

Majority of students have no problems with mouth taping and they breathe only through the nose during the whole night. Their mouth is not dry in the morning and they report numerous benefits of mouth taping. However, some students may find it difficult and uncomfortable so that they remove the tape during the night. These incidents have physiological causes, including:

1. Sleeping on the back. If you turn on your back during night sleep, your breathing gets almost twice heavier and it will be very difficult

to pump more air through the nose. Hence, learn the module devoted to prevention of sleeping on one's back.

2. Too warm sleep conditions. If your blanket is too warm, your breathing becomes deeper and bigger during sleep. You will wake up finding out that breathing through the nose is uncomfortable. To prevent overheating, use less warm clothes and blankets during sleep.

3. Carpets in your bedroom. Presence of carpets makes air quality tens or even hundreds times worse. During night sleep several cubic meters of air with millions of all these airborne particles, including dust, dust mites, their droppings, bacteria, viruses, etc. will enter through the nasal passages making them dryer and penetrating into bronchi and the lungs causing stress for the immune system and deep breathing. Sleeping in carpet-free rooms or covering carpets with plastic will solve this problem.

4. Very dusty pillow cases, blankets, and bed sheets create the same effect, as well as books, newspapers, hanging clothes, and old dusty curtains. Make sure that your bedroom has good air quality.

5. Closed windows during the night greatly worsen air quality in the bedroom due to poor air circulation and absence of air ions that make air cleaner. Either keep windows open or, if it is too cold or too noisy outside, buy an air ionizer/purifier and keep it running through the night.

6. Skin rashes due to extreme skin sensitivity. Try to find a hypoallergic tape or surgical paper tape. If rashes still a problem, you can sew together two clean socks making a circle. Wear it at night around your head so that to keep your jaw closed.

11.3 More ideas about nose breathing during the day

Some older people may use mouth taping during the day, if they have memory problems or can forget about the role of nasal breathing due to other factors.

If you have family members or friendly co-workers and you want to prevent mouth-breathing during the day, tell them that your doctor (Artour Rakhimov, PhD) prescribed you nasal breathing 24/7. Ask them to pay attention to the way you breathe and remind you about your commitment to solve this problem.

Use stickers on your PC screen, doors, desks, etc. reminding you, "Breathe only through the nose". Keep a large mirror on your working desk so that you can see your face and the way you breathe through.

If you have children, promise them a small treat if they catch you breathing through the mouth.

Nasal breathing during physical exercise will be very important. Always slow down or take rest if you exercise so intensively that you get a strong urge to open your mouth.

Your struggle will not be long. You should increase your morning CP up to 20 s or more. Hence, take care about other Modules so that to move up to the safe zone and get busy with more advanced challenges in your life and your Buteyko journey.

11.4 How to Prevent Sleeping on One's Back

First of all, if you have doubts about importance of sleeping positions or about prevention of sleeping on one's back, you can conduct a simple test described above in the Morning hyperventilation section. Measure your body oxygenation (the CP test) after sleeping in different sleeping positions. You can use an electrical clock with elimination showing seconds or a ticking mechanical clock so that there is no need to turn the light on. Note that you should spend about 10-15 minutes in a certain position in order to achieve a stable metabolism correspondent to this sleeping position. Sleeping on the back is worst and causes lowest body oxygenation.

If you find that your CP does not decrease (or maybe even improve) after sleeping on your back, you must sleep on the back all the time. However, none of Russian doctors ever met or heard about such people. Why?

According to Dr. Buteyko, *"Many severely sick patients remain sitting up, afraid to lie down. This is sensible. We should lie down only for a minimum amount of time, and only when sleeping. Our patients with deep breathing practice [breathing exercises], but cannot control their breathing at night, and hence, sleep is actually a poison for them. The longer he sleeps, the more chances that his breathing will be increased causing attacks. Therefore, we wake him up after 1-2 hours, he practices decreasing respiration...*

Children, especially asthmatics, or the deep-breathing children turn themselves over on the tummy during sleep. And here it begins: the parents are on guard, the fight goes on, sometimes for years. The child turns on the tummy hiding its head under the pillow, but no, they turn him over to face up. Again and again he tries to rescue [himself], but they will not give in. There is no rest for him, nor for the others. And if we take a child sick with asthma, he sleeps on his back and wheezes. He turned on his tummy, the wheezing disappears in a minute. [He is] again on his back: in a minute the wheezing starts again."

Sleeping on the back for many sick people means about twice as much breathing and corresponding CP drop. This often causes acute symptoms due to early morning hours and death in severely sick people. Hence, Dr. Buteyko, his medical colleagues who practiced the Buteyko breathing method, and their numerous patients used variety of tools to prevent sleeping on one's back. Let me list some of them.

1. Some people were sleeping with a backpack to prevent turning on the back. This is one ("awkward") option.

2. It is possible to prop oneself from the sides with pillows.

3. Another option is to sew a pocket on the back of your night shirt and put a tennis ball there.

4. Or one can take a sock and wrap it around the middle of a belt making a knot. The belt can be positioned around the middle of the chest with the knot on the back of the person. The knot should be big enough to prevent the person from sleeping on the back and it would not wake the person up since it is soft.

5. Currently, the most popular solution is to take a double cotton layer (strip) of bed linen about 2 m long and 20-30 cm wide. Wrap it around self, make two knots on your chest and move them on your back. A simple scarf can be also used.

Practice shows, that sleeping on the back is the sign of low CP. This problem is present when the CP is about 20 s or less. Once, your morning CP is over 25 s, you are very unlikely to sleep on your back at all and there is no need to use any of these techniques.

11.5 Your personal daily log

Main daily log for short Buteyko breathing sessions and for DIY breathing device sessions - 1 page (Rich-Text Format or PDF file or Excel Spreadsheet) All these links are on this page:
http://www.normalbreathing.com/free-downloads.php

About the author: Dr. Artour Rakhimov

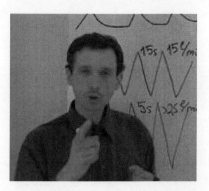

* High School Honor student (Grade "A" for all exams)
* Moscow University Honor student (Grade "A" for all exams)
* Moscow University PhD (Math/Physics), accepted in Canada and the UK
* Winner of many regional competitions in mathematics, chess and sport orienteering (during teenage and University years)
* Good classical piano-player: Chopin, Bach, Tchaikovsky, Beethoven, Strauss (up to now)
* Former captain of the ski-O varsity team and member of the cross-country skiing varsity team of the Moscow State University, best student teams of the USSR
* Former individual coach of world-elite athletes from Soviet (Russian) and Finnish national teams who took gold and silver medals during World Championships
* Total distance covered by running, cross country skiing, and swimming: over 100,000 km or over 2.5 loops around the Earth
* Joined Religious Society of Friends (Quakers) in 2001
* Author of the publication which won Russian National 1998 Contest of scientific and methodological sport papers
* Author of the books, as well as an <u>author of the bestselling Amazon books</u>:
  - *"Oxygenate Yourself: Breathe Less" (Buteyko Books; 94 pages; ISBN: 0954599683; 2008; Hardcover)*
  - *"<u>Cystic Fibrosis</u> Life Expectancy: 30, 50, 70, ..." 2012 - Amazon Kindle book*

- "Doctors Who Cure Cancer" *2012 - Amazon Kindle book*
- "Yoga Benefits Are in Breathing Less" *2012 - Amazon Kindle book*
- "Crohn's Disease and Colitis: Hidden Triggers and Symptoms" *2012 - Amazon Kindle book*
- "How to Use Frolov Breathing Device (Instructions)" *- 2012 - PDF and Amazon book (120 pages)*
- "Amazing DIY Breathing Device" *- 2010-2012 - PDF and Amazon book*
- *"What Science and Professor Buteyko Teach Us About Breathing" 2002*
- *"Breathing, Health and Quality of Life" 2004 (91 pages; Translated in Danish and Finnish)*
- *"Doctor Buteyko Lecture at the Moscow State University" 2009 (55 pages; Translation from Russian with Dr. A. Rakhimov's comments)*
- *"Normal Breathing: the Key to Vital Health" 2009 (The most comprehensive world's book on Buteyko breathing retraining method; over 190,000 words; 305 pages)*

* Author of the world's largest website devoted to breathing, breathing techniques, and breathing retraining (www.NormalBreathing.com)

* Author of numerous YouTube videos (http://www.youtube.com/user/artour2006)

* Buteyko breathing teacher (since 2002 up to now) and trainer

* Inventor of the Amazing DIY breathing device and numerous contributions to breathing retraining

* Whistleblower and investigator of mysterious murder-suicides, massacres and other crimes organized worldwide by GULAG KGB agents using the fast total mind control method

* Practitioner of the New Decision Therapy and Kantillation

* Level 2 Trainer of the New Decision Therapy

* Health writer and health educator